The Healthy Family Cookbook

89+1 Delicious Recipes to Help Prevent and Reverse Disease for the Whole Family

Oliver Gundry

DIABETIC DESSERT COOKBOOK

Diabetic and Prediabetic Guilt Free Guide to Prepare Delicious Low carb and Low Sugar Desserts, Cookies, Bread and Cakes that Whole Family Can Enjoy for Healthy Sweet Moments

By Oliver Gundry

Introduction

Maintaining a healthy weight is vital for everyone, but if you have diabetes, excess weight can make your blood sugar levels more difficult to control and may increase your risk of some complications. Weight loss can be an extra challenge for people with diabetes. You need to eat healthily as you seek to lose weight, but if you have diabetes, eating the wrong diet may harm your health. Pills for weight loss and diets for malnutrition can be avoided at every cost but several common diets can be helpful.

You must focus on consuming lean protein, fewer carbs, and no processed food, high-fiber, fruits and vegetables, dairy with low fat, or if you can find it fat-free, and healthy vegetable fats such as nuts, avocado, olive oil or canola oil if you have diabetes. Your food consumption will be handled as well. Having your doctor or dietitian have meals and snacks with a specific carb level. In total, women should be aiming about 45 grams of carb per meal and men should be aiming 60. It will preferably come from dynamic grains, nuts, and vegetables.

The American Diabetes Association offers a detailed guide regarding the best foods for people with diabetes. The recommendations include:

Proteins: beans, eggs, poultry, nuts, and salmon, sardines, and tuna.

Dairy: non-fat or low-fat yogurt and non-fat or low-fat yogurt.

Fruits/Vegetables: sweet potatoes, berries, and okra, kale, asparagus, and broccoli.

Grains such as whole wheat pasta, whole grains; brown rice.

Staying hydrated is critical in terms of physical safety, too. Whenever necessary choose non-caloric alternatives such as water and tea.

Chapter 1. Kinds of Diets Good for Prediabetic or Diabetic Persons

Certain foods should be limited to people with diabetes. These foods may trigger blood sugar spikes or contain harmful fats.

They cover:

- Grains cooked, for example, white rice or white pasta

- Introduced sweetening foods, including apple sauce, jelly, and some canned foods

- Full-fat dairy

- Products fried or heavy in trans fats or saturated fats

- Products produced from fine wheat

- Every product that has a heavy glycemic value

1. The dietary approach to stop hypertension (DASH) plan

Originally intended to better manage or avoid high blood pressure (hypertension), the DASH program may also decrease the likelihood of certain diseases, also diabetes. This will even have the additional advantage of helping you drop weight. People who follow the DASH diet are encouraged to reduce portion sizes and eat foods rich in nutrients that lower blood pressure, such as potassium, magnesium, and calcium.

The DASH meal program contains:

- Protein lean: Fish, Poultry

- Foods based on plants: vegetables, fruits, beans, nuts, seeds

- Dairy items: animal goods free of fat or reduced in fat

- Whole grains

- Healthy fats: Oils from vegetables

In this program, it is advised that people with diabetes limit their sodium consumption to 1,500 milligrams a day. The program even bans chocolate, sugary drinks, and red meats.

2. The Mediterranean diet

This diet is influenced by typical Mediterranean diets. This diet is rich in oleic acid, a fatty acid naturally present in fats and oils based on animals and vegetables. Countries known to eat from this diet include Greece, Italy, and Morocco.

According to research in Diabetes Spectrum, a Mediterranean-type diet may be effective in reducing glucose levels, lowering body weight, and lowering the risk of metabolic disorder.

Foods eaten during this diet shall include:

• Protein: salmon, poultry, fried fish and other species

• Food dependent on plants: fruit, vegetables such as artichokes and cucumbers, beans, nuts, seeds

• Good fats: coconut oil, almond nuts,

Red meat can be eaten once a month. Alcohol should be drunk in moderation because it can improve cardiac safety. Remember you should never drink when you have an empty stomach if you are on medicines that increase insulin levels in your body.

3. The Paleolithic Diet

This diet focuses on the assumption that the responsibility for chronic disease rests with modern agriculture. Paleo diet adherents consume only that which our ancient ancestors may have hunted and harvested.

Foods consumed during the Paleo diet include:

• Protein: meat, fish, poultry,

• Non-starchy foods: grains, fruits, seeds, nuts (excluding peanuts)

• Balanced fats: walnut oil, avocado oil, olive oil, coconut oil, flaxseed oil

A paleo diet is a good option for persons with diabetes as long as the person has fine and healthy kidneys. A paleo diet can boost glycemic regulation in the short term for people with type 2 diabetes, according to a three-month analysis reported in the Journal of Diabetes Science and Technology.

4. Vegan or Vegetarian Diets

Any diabetes sufferers focus on consuming a vegetarian diet. Vegetarian diets usually apply to diets where no meat is consumed, but may contain animal items such as milk, poultry, or butter. Vegan individuals do not consume beef or other food items, including honey, butter, or gelatin.

Foods that are healthy for vegetarians and vegans with diabetes include:

• Soy

• Fruits

• Beans

• Leafy vegetables

• Legumes

• Nuts

- Whole grains

Although vegan or vegetarian diets can be healthier diets to adopt, if not vigilant, those that pursue them might be losing out on crucial nutrients.

Some nutrients vegans or vegetarians might need to consume using supplements include:

- Iodine. The iodine required to metabolize food into energy is contained primarily
- in seafood. Without these animal items, vegetarians or vegans may have difficulty having enough of the requisite iodine in their diets. Supplements, however, can help.
- Zinc: The primary supply of zinc is from high protein meat foods, so anyone with a vegetarian diet will be recommended to provide a replacement.
- Calcium. Calcium found mainly in animal products such as dairy, is an essential nutrient that contributes greatly to bone and teeth health. Kale or broccoli may help provide the calcium required, although a vegan diet may require supplements.
- B-12: Because only animal products have vitamin B-12, anyone adopting a strict vegetarian diet will need to use a supplement.

5. Gluten-free diet

Gluten-free diets have been common but the removal of gluten from the diet is important for people with celiac disease to prevent harm to the colon and body. Celiac disease is an autoimmune disorder that triggers an attack on your gut and nervous system by your immune system. It also causes inflammation in the body and may contribute to chronic disease.

Gluten is a nutrient present in maize, rye, barley, and other grain products. 10 percent of people with type 1 diabetes often have celiac disease, according to the American Diabetes Association.

Tell the doctor to perform a celiac disorder blood check. You may also be intolerant of gluten even though it falls low. Talk to your doctor about whether you should have a gluten-free diet.

While anyone with diabetes may take a gluten-free diet, it may introduce restrictions for anyone without the celiac disease. Recalling that gluten-free is not equated with low carb, too. Processed, high-sugar products that are gluten-free are available. There's usually no such need to make meal planning complicated by eradicating gluten until you need it.

Physical activity is important for the wellbeing of people with diabetes in addition to having the correct diet. Exercise can help to reduce rates of blood sugar and A1C and may help to prevent risks.

Even if you see improvement with physical exercise, don't change your prescribed insulin routine without your doctor's advice. If you are taking insulin and trying to add or implementing adjustments to your fitness routine, test before, during, and after exercise. This is true even if you think the weight gain is caused by the insulin. Changing your insulin schedule could affect your blood sugar levels. These modifications may trigger problems that could endanger life.

If you're worried about your weight, speak to a doctor or nutritionist. They will help you choose the lifestyle that fits your unique dietary requirements and expectations for weight loss. They can also help avoid food and drug problems and can interfere with prescription drugs.

Chapter 2. Recipes for Low-Carb and Low-Sugar Desserts, Cookies, Cakes, Bread and More

A healthy diabetic diet is all about equilibrium. As long as moderation is taken into account, the total amount of carbohydrates in your diet makes up a small amount of sugar. As a general rule, diabetics will seek to cut down on products and beverages that contain high levels of sugar as they can find it more difficult to regulate blood sugar and weight. If you adopt a diabetic diet, these smaller, safer treats are good sweets to think. All of these 45 dishes are around 30 g or fewer carbs per meal.

1. Cream Cheese Brownies

It takes 20 minutes for preparation and 25 minutes for baking. You can make 1 dozen brownies with the following ingredients.

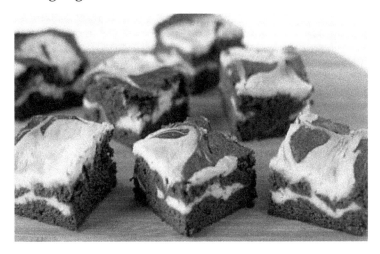

- Large eggs (3)
- Soft, low-fat Butter (6 tablespoons)
- Sugar; 1 cup
- Half cup flour (all-purpose)
- Baking cocoa; ¼ cup
- Low-fat cream cheese; 8 oz. 1 Packet

Preheat the oven to 350 ° C. Set aside 2 eggs separately, place each white in a bowl (save for later use). Beat butter and 3/4 cup sugar in a small bowl, until crumbly. Beat 1 egg white and vanilla in the remaining whole egg until well combined. Combine the flour and cocoa; slowly transfer until combined to the egg mixture. Pour into a 9 inches square pan for baking. Line the pan with cooking spray; set away.

Beat the remaining sugar and the cream cheese in a bowl, until smooth. Beat white in the second shell. Fall into the batter by rounded tablespoonfuls; slash into the batter to churn with a knife.

Bake for 25 to 30 minutes or until complete, then take the edges from the sides of the plate. Cool it down on a rack of string.

2. Tiramisu Cake

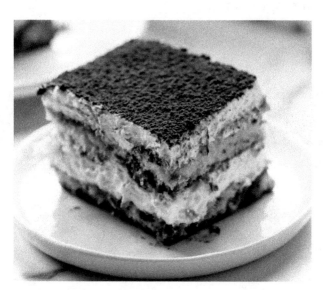

This cake requires 25-30 minutes for preparation. You can easily prepare 9 servings with these ingredients.

- Baking cocoa
- Ladyfinger cookies (24)
- Heavy cream; Half cup
- Vanilla yogurt; 2 cups
- Fat-free or low-fat milk; 1 cup

- Strong coffee or espresso; Half cup

- Raspberries (optional)

Beat the cream in a small bowl until it gets stiff; fold yogurt. Place 1/2 cup cream mixture over an 8 inches dish.

Mix the milk and espresso into a shallow dish. Dip 12 ladyfingers into the coffee mixture quickly, allowing excess drip away. Set in a single layer in the dish, breaking to fit as required. Fill with half the remaining milk mixture; cocoa wax. Repeat across walls.

Cap, refrigerate, at least 2 hours before eating. Serve with raspberries if you prefer.

3. Ginger Plum Tart

This tart requires a total of 35 to 40 minutes including preparation, baking, and cooling. It makes up to 8 servings.

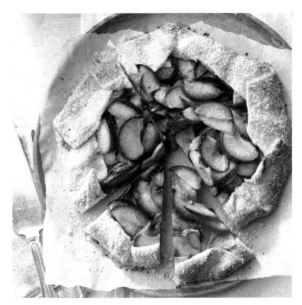

- Large egg (1) only egg white

- Pie crust (refrigerated)

- Fresh plums (sliced); 3 and a half cups

- Coarse sugar (1 teaspoon and 3 tablespoons)

- Cornstarch; 1 tablespoon

- Crystallized ginger (chopped); 2 teaspoons

- Water; 1 tablespoon

Preheat the oven to 400°. Unroll crust on a work surface. Then roll it in a 12-inches circle. Transfer to a baking sheet covered with parchment.

Toss the plums in a wide bowl with 3 spoonsful of cornstarch and sugar. Arrange crust plums up to about 2 in. Of the edges; sprinkle the ginger over. Fold the edge of the crust

over the prunes and pleat as you go.

Whisk egg white and water in a small bowl; sprinkle over folded crust. Sprinkle of extra sugar.

Bake for 20 to 25 minutes, until crust is golden brown. Cool on a wire rack, on a tray. Serve warm, or at ambient temperature.

4. Cake - Pear Bundt

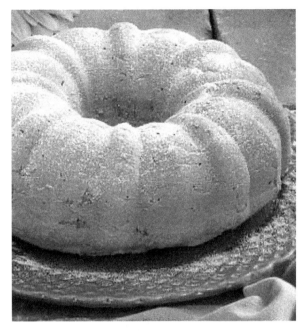

The cake gives you around 15 to 16 servings using the following ingredients. Moreover, it takes about one hour including preparation, baking, and cooling.

- Sliced pears (sugar reduced) 1 can

- White cake mix; 1 Packet

- Large eggs (2) egg whites only

- Large egg; 1, whole

- Confectioner sugar; 2 teaspoons

Drain pears and set aside the syrup; chop pears. In a big cup, put the pears and syrup; add the cake mixture, the egg whites, and the butter. Beat 30 seconds on low speed. Beat 4 minutes on high.

Coat them in a 10-inches tube pan with cooking spray and flour residue. Add the ingredients.

Bake at 350 ° until 50 to 55 minutes comes out clean with a toothpick inserted in the middle. Give it 10 minutes to cool completely before transferring from pan to wire rack. Dust it using the confectioner sugar.

However, you can use other fruits as well as frozen strawberries with a white cake mix to work well!

5. Banana Raspberry Soft Serve (ice cream)

The total time this soft serve takes is around 10 to 15 minutes plus cooling. The following ingredients can make 2 cups easily.

- Ripe bananas; 4 medium-sized
- Fat-free yogurt; Half cup
- Maple syrup; 1 to 2 tablespoons
- Unsweetened Raspberries (frozen); Half cup
- Raspberries/blueberries (fresh); optional

Thinly slice the bananas; transfer to something like a large plastic resealable freezer bag. Set slices together in a layer and then freeze them overnight.

Pulse the bananas until finely diced in a food processor. Add milk, raspberries and maple syrup. Then process until smooth, scrubbing sides as necessary. Serve straight away, add fresh berries if you wish.

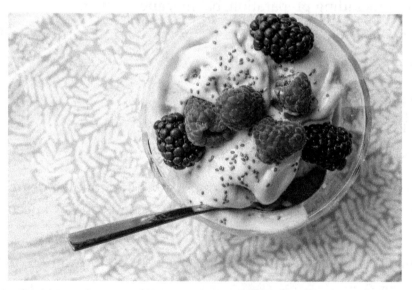

Chocolate-Peanut Butter: Substitute for the raspberries; 2 tablespoons of each peanut butter or baking cocoa; continue as instructed.

6. Butterscotch Pumpkin Gingerbread Trifle

It requires 40 minutes for preparation and baking requires around 35 to 40 minutes. Cooling takes extra time. It makes up to 16 servings.

- Gingerbread cookie or cake mix (1 packet)
- Fat-free or low-fat milk; 4 cups
- Ground cinnamon (1 teaspoon)
- Butterscotch pudding (sugar-free) mix; 4 packets 1 oz. each
- Ground ginger; ¼ teaspoon
- Ground allspice; ¼ teaspoon
- Ground nutmeg; ¼ teaspoon
- Pumpkin; 1 can, 15 oz.
- Whipped topping (low-fat, frozen) 12 oz.

Prepare and bake the gingerbread mix according to cake packaging directions. Then, cool it.

Break the cake into crumbles; save the crumbs for 1/4 cup. Whisk the butter, pudding mixtures, and spices in a wide bowl until the mixture thickens, around 2 minutes. Stir in the pumpkin.

In a qt of 3–1/2. trifle or glass cup, 1/4 layer of cake crumbs, 1/2 pumpkin mixture, 1/4 of the cake crumbs, and 1/2 whipped topping; repeat the layering. Top with crumbs that are reserved. Chill once done.

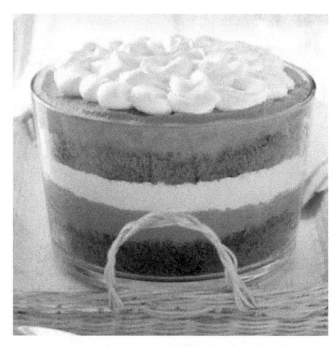

7. Raspberry Chocolate Cheesecake

This cheesecake takes around 25 to 30 minutes for preparation then it takes some time to cool off. You can prepare 12 servings using the following ingredients.

- Melted butter; 2 tablespoons

- Crumbs of Graham Crackers; ¾ cup

- Gelatin (unflavored); 1 envelope

- Coldwater; 1 cup

- Half cup sugar

- Baking cocoa; ¼ cup

- Semisweet chocolate (chopped); 4 oz.

- Cream cheese (fat-free or low-fat); 4 packets 8 oz. each

- Vanilla extract; 2 teaspoons

- Fresh raspberries; 2 cups

- Sugar substitute; 1 cup sugar

Combine cracker crumbs and butter; push to a grated 9 inches pan. Bake for 8-10 minutes at 375 °, or until light brown. Cool it off.

Sprinkle the gelatin over cold water in a medium saucepan for filling; let stand for 1 minute. Heat over low heat, stirring until the gelatin dissolves completely. Stir in the semi-sweet candy, once cooled.

Beat the cream cheese, sugar replacement, and butter in a large bowl until they are smooth. Gradually substitute the blend of sugar and cocoa. Fill them in coffee. Pour over the crust; cool for 2-3 hours or until solid.

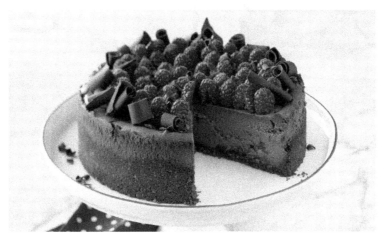

Set raspberries on a cheesecake. Loosen the cake from the pan using a knife carefully.

8. Chocolate chip cookies – Browned Butter

Butter shifts from nutty and sweet to salty and easily charred, but make careful to remove the pan from the fire until it becomes amber-colored. Make sure the cookie sheet is absolutely clean before beginning the next batch to prevent cookies from spreading.

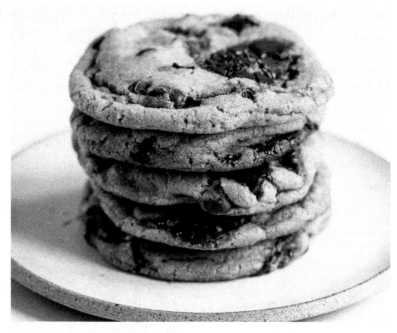

- Unsalted Butter; 6 tablespoons

- Canola oil; 2 tablespoons

- All-purpose flour; 5.6 oz.

- Whole-wheat flour; 3.3 oz.

- Baking powder; 1 teaspoon

- Kosher salt; Half teaspoon

- Brown sugar; ¾ cup

- Granulated sugar; 2/3 cup

- Vanilla extract; Half teaspoon

- Large eggs (2), slightly beaten

- Chocolate chips (semisweet); Half cup

- Hershey's Chocolate chips (dark); 1/3 cup

Preheat the oven to 375°.

Heat the butter over medium heat in a small saucepan; cook for 5 minutes or until brown. Take off heat; add oil. Put aside to freshen up.

Weigh or gently spoon flours into dry cups of measurement; level with a knife. Stir with a fork, mix flours, baking powder, and salt. Put the butter and sugar mixture in a bowl; beat at medium speed with a mixer until mixed. Add eggs and vanilla; beat till it's blended. Add flour mixture, beat at low velocity until just mixed. Add chocolate chips.

Pour 2 inches on baking trays lined with a waxed paper by even spoonful. Bake for 12 minutes or when cookie bottoms only start to get brown. Then cool them a bit.

9. Chocolate Coconut Cupcakes

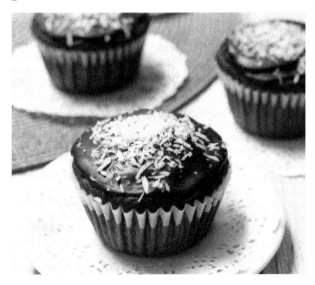

These cupcakes require 20 minutes for preparation, 30 minutes for baking, and then some time to cool off. You can make around a dozen cupcakes.

- Egg whites (large eggs); 6
- All-purpose flour; 2/3 cup
- Baking cocoa; ¼ cup
- Baking powder; Half teaspoon
- Sugar; 1 to 1 1/3 cup
- Almond extract; 1 teaspoon
- Cream of tartar; 1 teaspoon
- Salt; ¼ teaspoon

- Shredded Coconut (sweetened); 1 cup
- Confectioner Sugar

Preheat your oven to 350°.

Put the egg whites in a bowl. Line 18 cups of cupcake muffin liners. Mix the flour, baking powder, cocoa, and 1 cup of sugar.

Add almond extract, tartar cream, and salt to egg whites; beat at medium velocity until soft peaks develop. Gradually add the remaining sugar, 1 teaspoon at a time, and beat before the sugar is dissolved. Continue to beat until stiff glittering peaks emerge. Gradually add in flour mixture, one and a half cup at a time. Fold softly in a cocoon.

Fill two-thirds of prepared cups completely. Bake for 30 to 35 minutes, until the top is crisp.

Wait in pans for 10 minutes before transferring to wire racks; cool the cupcakes completely. Dust it off using confectioner sugar if needed.

10. Apple Pie (No Bake)

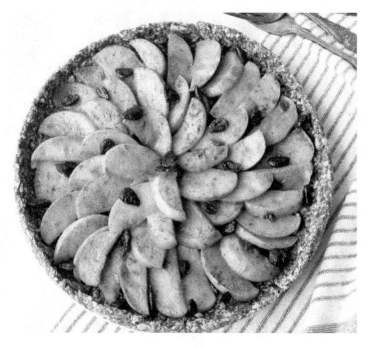

Apples are distributed often during the year and that is something you should take advantage of. This pie takes about 20-25 minutes for preparation. Then, it takes time to cool off. The following ingredients can prepare up to 8 servings.

- Tart apples; medium-sized; 5; sliced and peeled
- Lemon gelatin (sugar-free); 1 packet
- Ground cinnamon; Half teaspoon
- Ground nutmeg; ¼ teaspoon
- Water (divided); 1 and ¾ cups
- Sugar-free Vanilla Pudding mix
- Chopped Nuts; Half cup
- Crust made using Graham Crackers; 1 piece
- Whipped topping

Mix the gelatin, nutmeg, cinnamon, and water in a large saucepan. Stir in apples; put to a simmer. Reduce heat; boil, cover, for around 5 minutes, until apples are tender.

Mix pudding mixture and remaining water in a bowl; stir in apple mixture. Cook for about 1 minute, stirring occasionally until thickened. Take off heat; stir in the nuts. Remove it from the pan.

Refrigerate the pie two hours before eating. Serve with whipped topping if desired.

11. Frozen Yogurt and Berry Popsicle Swirls

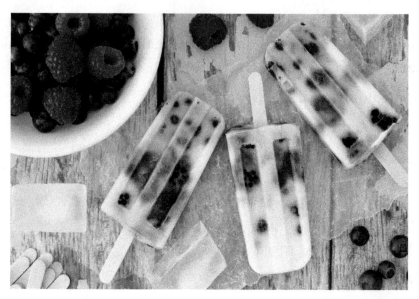

Preparation for these swirls requires 15 to 20 minutes. It is a good and healthy way to ease your ice cream or sugar cravings. After preparation, it takes time to freeze. You can make 10 popsicles with the following ingredients.

- Fresh berries; 1 cup
- Fat-free Greek Yogurt; 2 ¾ cups
- Paper or Plastic cups; 10
- Water; ¼ cup
- Sugar; 2 tablespoons
- Pop sticks (wooden); 10

Every cup is filled with around 1/4 cup yogurt. In a food processor, put the berries, water, and sugar; pulse until the berries are finely chopped. spoon berry mixture into each cup. Stir softly and play with a pop button.

Foil the cups from the top; drop through foil the pop sticks. Freeze them until they are solid.

For Frozen Yogurt Clementine Swirls: Replace 1 cup of clementine seeded segments and 1/4 cup of orange juice for sugar, berries, and water; follow the instructions.

12. Root Beer Pie

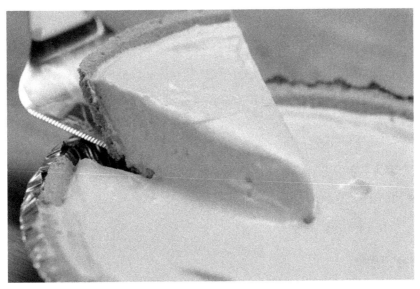

For its preparation, you will need 15 to 20 minutes. You need the following ingredients for this pie.

- Crust; Graham Cracker
- Vanilla Pudding Mix; 1 packet
- Whipped topping (low-fat); frozen
- Diet root beer; ¾ cup
- Fat-free or low-fat milk; Half cup
- Cherries (optional)

Set aside and cool for garnish the whipped coating. Whisk the root beer, sugar, and pudding mixture in a wide bowl for 2 minutes. Fold the leftover whipped topping in two. Apply on the crust of graham cracker.

Place over tar left whipped coating. Freeze at least eight hours, or overnight.

Garnish the reserved whipped topping over each serving; if desired, top with a cherry maraschino.

13. Jelly and Peanut Butter Sandwich Cookies

Peanut butter cookies form the ideal basis for spreading a coating of delicious strawberry. Serve some delicious cookies as an afternoon snack or a surprise warm lunchbox.

- Soft margarine; ¼ cup

- Peanut butter (creamy); no sugar; ¼ cup

- Sweetener (calorie-free); Half cup

- Sugar; ¼ cup

- Egg whites (2); Large eggs

- Vanilla Extract; 1 teaspoon

- All-purpose Flour; 1 ¾ cup

- Baking soda; 1 teaspoon

- Salt, 1/8 teaspoon

- Cooking spray

- Strawberry spread (low-sugar); ¾ cup

Preheat the oven to 350°.

Beat peanut butter and butter until creamy, with a mixer at medium speed. Gradually add sugar and sweetener, and beat well. Then add the vanilla and the egg whites. In a bowl, combine the flour, salt, and soda, and stir well. Gradually add the flour to the creamed mixture and beat well.

Dough form into 40 balls, 1-inch each. Put the balls with a distance of 2 inches between them on cooking spray-coated baking sheets. Use a glass or anything flat to flatten the cookies into 2-inch circles. Bake for 8 to 9 minutes at 350 °, or until lightly browned. Cool on pans; cut, and let cool down on wire racks.

Spread strawberry on each of the 20 cookies at the bottom; top with remaining cookies.

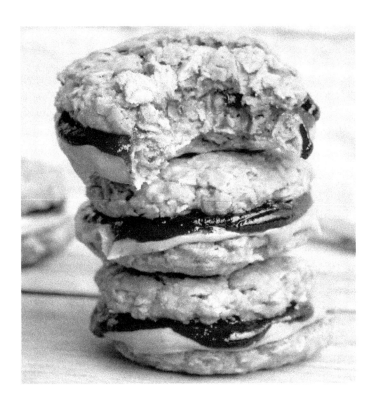

14. Pudding Pie

For someone with diabetes, this pie is surely what you need to quench your sugar cravings. It takes 20 minutes for preparation. You can make 8 servings using the

following ingredients.

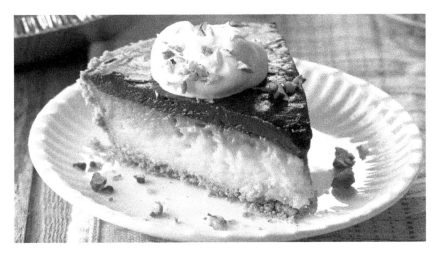

- Fat-free milk; 4 cups

- Vanilla pudding mix; 1 oz. (sugar-free)

- Crust; Graham Cracker

- Butterscotch pudding mix; 1 oz. (sugar-free)

- Chocolate pudding mix; 1 oz. (sugar-free)

- Whipped topping

- Chopped pecans

Whisk the milk and the vanilla pudding mixture for 2 minutes. Spread over crust.

Whisk butterscotch pudding mixture and milk in another bowl for 2 minutes. Carefully spoon over the top of the coffee, thinly distributed.

Whisk the remaining 1-1/3 cups of milk and chocolate pudding mixture into a separate bowl for 2 minutes. Spread carefully over top. Refrigerate at least 30 minutes when you are done. Serve with whipped toppings and pecans if needed.

15. Chocolate Cupcakes

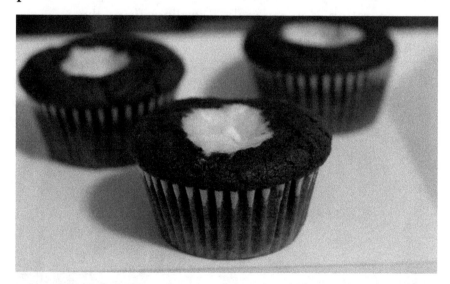

Inside these chocolate cupcakes is a secret, delicious filling of coconut and ricotta cheese. These cupcakes require 20 minutes for preparation and around 30 minutes for baking. Then, it takes time to cool off. You can make a dozen cupcakes with the following ingredients.

- Egg whites; 2 large eggs

- Large egg (1)

- Applesauce (unsweetened); 1/3 cup

- Vanilla extract; 1 teaspoon

- All-purpose flour; 1 to 1 ¼ cups

- Sugar; 1 cup

- Baking cocoa; 1/3 cup

- Baking soda; ½ teaspoon

- Buttermilk; ¾ cup

To prepare the filling for the cupcakes, you need:

- Ricotta cheese (low-fat); 1 cup

- Sugar; ¼ cup

- Egg white; 1 large egg

- Shredded coconut (sweetened); 1/3 cup

- Almond or coconut extract; Half teaspoon

- Confectioner Sugar

Preheat your oven to 350°. Coat 18 muffin cups with cooking oil.

Beat 4 ingredients first, until well combined. Whisk together flour, cocoa, sugar, and baking soda in another bowl; slowly beat alternately with buttermilk into an egg mixture.

Beat the ricotta cheese, sugar, and white egg until combined for filling. Stir in coconut.

Fill the muffin cups using batter but use only half. Fill your filling into the middle of each cupcake by the tablespoonfuls; cover with remaining batter.

Bake for 28 to 33 minutes and wait for the toothpick inserted in the cupcake to come out neat. Transfer after 10 minutes on wire racks before removing from the pans. Dust it using confectioners' sugar.

15. Wheat and Seed Bread

This bread is expensive to make than normal loaves of bread, so for a couple of days, I recommend you slice and freeze any that you won't use. Despite the high fat and protein content, it is full. I don't need insulin for that sandwich, but it's not the same for everybody. For anything that includes a touch of carbohydrate, I require insulin so I realized that the protein and fat in the ingredients would help offset the carbohydrates in

the ingredients, but I was also happily shocked that I didn't need insulin at all. No sugar, no hypo- threat. This bread is good not only for people with diabetes but for everyone.

- Almond flour; 80 grams
- Coconut flour; 30 grams
- Psyllium Husk; 20 grams
- Melted Butter; 30 grams
- Buttermilk; 1 cup
- Mixed seeds
- Baking powder; ¼ teaspoon
- Bread soda; Half teaspoon
- Flaxseed; 50 grams
- Wheat Bran; 30 grams

Preheat your oven to 180°C. Line a one-pound loaf tin with baking parchment paper or you can also use a liner if you want.

Sieve into a cup the coconut and almond or ground almond, bread soda, and baking powder. Add the rest of the dry ingredients, also the seeds.

Combine the buttermilk, eggs and melted butter in a bowl, then mix.

Build a well with the dry ingredients in the middle. Add the liquid and stir to mix both the dry ingredients and the liquid in a circular motion. Don't over-mix them. A loose batter is what you need as your mixture.

Put your mixture into a lined loaf pan. Place first 15 minutes in the preheated oven, then lower it to 150 ° C. Bake for another 25 minutes or until the bread is baked. You will see the bread rising from the edges of the pan. The time taken to cook depends on your oven.

Allow the bread to cool on a rack. The bread can be kept for 3 to 4 days in the freezer, although the day it is cooked it needs to be frozen if you decide to preserve it longer.

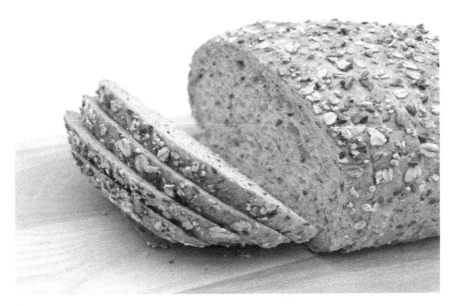

16. Coffee Cupcakes

Such chocolatey cupcakes are kept on the lighter side using low-fat whipped icing to dust them. You should substitute the prune puree with unsweetened applesauce if you want.

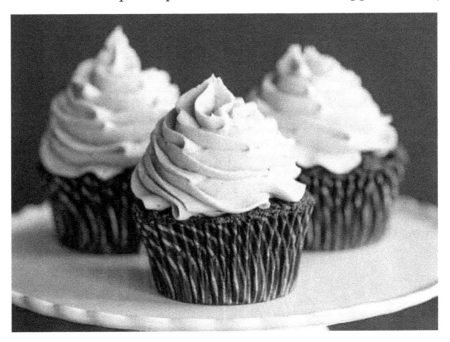

It takes about 15 minutes for preparation. For baking, the cupcakes need 20 minutes. Then, cooling requires extra time!

- Eggs (2)

- All-purpose flour; 2 cups

- Baking cocoa; Half cup

- Baking soda; 1 teaspoon

- Salt; Half teaspoon

- Hot water; Half cup

- Coffee Granules (instant); ¼ cup

- Baby food; Half cup

- Canola oil; ¼ cup

- Vanilla extract; 2 teaspoons

- Whipped topping (low-fat)

- Baking cocoa (additional)

Combine the cocoa, flour, baking soda, sugar, and salt in a bowl. Dissolve the coffee in hot water. Whisk the whites, baby meal, butter, espresso, and coffee mixture in a big pot. Gradually mix in dry ingredients until moist.

Fill up two-thirds muffin cups. Bake for 18 to 20 minutes at 350 °, or until a toothpick comes out clean. Wait for about 10 minutes and then you can remove the cupcakes from pans to wire racks.

Shortly before eating, brush with chocolate and fill cupcakes with whipped icing. Store the leftovers in a refrigerator.

17. Chocolate Banana Cake

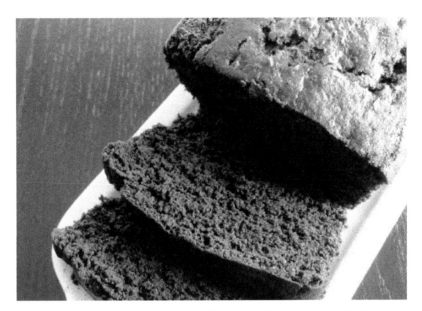

This chocolate light-as-air cake has a yummy banana flavor. It's delicious as it is, so you can dress it up with nuts or soft frostings as well. The cake requires 15 minutes for the preparation. It takes 25 minutes for baking and then it cools down. This cake has about 12 servings.

- Soft butter; 1/3 cup
- Sugar substitute; ¾ cup
- Brown sugar; 1/3 cup
- Vanilla extract; 2 teaspoons
- Large eggs (2)
- Water; Half cup
- All-purpose flour; 1 1/3 cup
- Milk powder (zero fat); Half cup
- Baking cocoa; 3 tablespoons
- Baking powder; 1 teaspoon
- Baking soda; Half teaspoon
- Salt; Half teaspoon
- Ripe bananas; mashed; 1 cup

- Confectioner sugar

Preheat the oven to 375°. Coat a 9 inches square pan using cooking spray.

Mix butter, a substitute for sugar, and brown sugar until light and fluffy. Then add the coffee and whites, beat well as you add each ingredient, one at a time. Stir the water in. Whisk together flour, cocoa, milk powder, baking soda, baking powder, and salt. Keep it mixing until you get a creamy texture. Stir in the bananas.

Switch to the prepared pan. Then bake for 23- to minutes before a toothpick inserted in the middle comes out clean and the cake starts to fall from the sides of the oven. Cool down on a wire rack. Dust it with confectioners' sugar.

18. Sour Cream Cake

This is a lighter cake recipe with the traditional one's flavor. Reduced-fat sour cream, without too many calories, contains moisture and flavor.

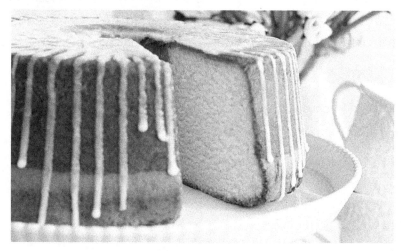

- Large eggs (3)
- Cooking spray
- Breadcrumbs; 3 tablespoons
- Cake flour; 4 cups
- Salt; ¼ teaspoon
- Sour cream (light); 1 and a half cup
- Baking soda; 1 teaspoon

- Butter; ¾ cup
- Sugar; 2 ¾ cups
- Vanilla extract; 2 teaspoons
- Lemon juice (fresh); 2 tablespoons

Preheat the oven to 350°.

Coat a 10 inches pan using cooking spray and dust it with breadcrumbs.

Lightly add flour in dry cups and level them using a knife. Combine flour and salt; mix with a whisk. Bring sour cream and baking soda together; stir well. Layer butter in a wide bowl; beat medium-speed using a mixer until light and fluffy. Gradually incorporate cinnamon and sugar, and beat until well combined. Remove whites, 1 at a time, then beat well with any addition. Then add some juice; beat for 30 seconds. Now, add flour mixture to sugar mixture, mixing at a low level, starting and finishing with flour mixture, and with the mixture of sour cream.

Spoon batter in ready pan. Bake for 1 hour and 10 minutes at 350 °, or until a center inserted wooden pick comes out clean. Cool for 10 minutes and then remove it from the pan. Fully cool on rack wire.

19. Crackle Cookies

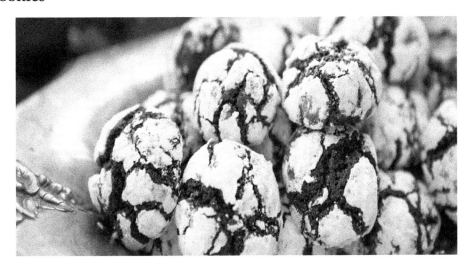

Without any guilt, you should treat yourself to one or two of those crackle cookies. It takes 20 minutes for preparation. And you can easily make 2 dozen cookies using the following ingredients.

- Sugar; 2/3 cup

- Large egg (1)

- Canola oil; ¼ cup

- Molasses; 1/3 cup

- Whole-wheat flour; 2 cups

- Baking soda; 1 teaspoon

- Ground cinnamon; 1 teaspoon

- Ground ginger; ¼ teaspoon

- Ground cloves; ¼ teaspoon

- Salt; Half teaspoon

- Confectioner Sugar; 1 tablespoon

Beat oil and sugar in a bowl, until mixed. Place in molasses and eggs. Combine the starch, baking soda, salt, cinnamon, cloves, and ginger; introduce the sugar mixture slowly, and blend properly. Refrigerate and cover for at least 2 hours.

Preheat the oven to 350°. Dough to 1-inch balls; roll the balls in confectioner sugar. Place the balls with 2 inches distance between them on a spray-coated baking sheet; partially flatten. Bake for seven to nine minutes or until completed. To cool off, place it on wire racks.

A single cookie contains approx. 77 calories.

20. Pudding Cookie Sandwiches

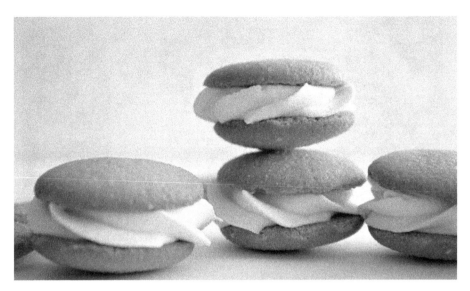

Preparation for these cookies requires 20 minutes. You can make more than 2 dozen cookies with the following ingredients.

- Fat-free or low-fat milk; 1 to 2 cups
- Chocolate pudding mix; sugar-free; 1.4 oz.
- Whipped topping; low-fat; frozen; 8 oz.
- Marshmallows; 1 cup
- Chocolate wafers; 9 oz.

Whisk the milk and pudding mix for 2 minutes to fill; allow it to stand for 2 minutes. Fold in topping and then marshmallows.

Place around 2 tablespoons onto the bottom of a wafer for each sandwich; cover with another wafer. Place the sandwiches in sealed pots.

Freeze up for around 3 hours. Remove from the freezer before 5 minutes to serve.

21. Chocolate Hazelnut Popsicles

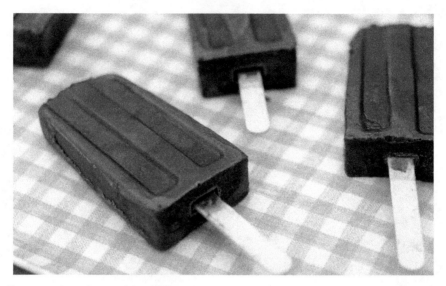

If you love Nutella as I do, this is the thing for you. You need 10 minutes for the preparation of these popsicles. And you can make 8 of these using the following ingredients.

- Nutella; 1/3 cup

- Popsicle molds or paper/plastic cups; 8

- Soy milk (vanilla); 1 cup

- Fat-free milk; Half cup

- Greek yogurt (vanilla) fat-free; ¾ cup

- Pop sticks (wooden)

Place Nutella, yogurt, and milk in a blender; cover it and blend it until smooth. Pour into paper cups or popsicle molds. Cover the molds with holders. If you are using cups, cover with foil and then insert sticks through the foil. Freeze until solid.

One popsicle contains approx. 94 to 95 calories.

22. Chocolate Cheesecake

This cheesecake appears indulgent, it is a lightened-up variety so you should feel confident about feeding your mates. It takes 30 minutes for preparation and 40 minutes for baking. The cooling time in between is extra. You can get 12 servings per cake.

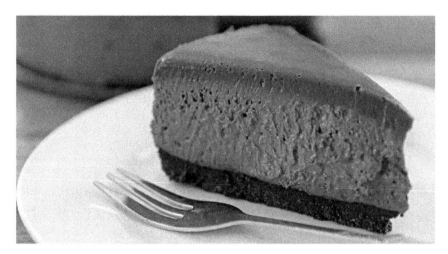

- Cottage Cheese; 2%; 2 cups

- Chocolate wafers (crushed); 1 cup

- Low-fat cream cheese; 1 packet; 8 oz.

- Sugar; Half cup

- Dash salt

- Vanilla extract; 1 tablespoon

- Large eggs (2); slightly beaten

- Egg white (1); a large egg

- Melted then cooled bittersweet chocolate; 2 oz.

- Raspberries are optional

Fill a strainer with cheesecloth having four layers or a coffee filter; position it over a pot. Put the cottage cheese in a strainer; refrigerate for 1 hour. Bring in a 9 inches pan at a double thickness of foil, tightly seal foil around the pan. Coat with a cooking spray inside of the pan. Push down broken wafers, then 1-inch to the upper side.

Preheat the oven to 350°. Process drained cheese in a food processor until it is smooth. Attach cinnamon, sugar, and cream cheese; heat until combined. Shift to a bowl and then add the egg white, eggs, and coffee. In a bowl, remove 1 cup batter; mix in molten chocolate.

Drop the batter on your crust. Place chocolate cake over simple batter. Cut with a knife to run into water. Transfer to a bigger pan. Then add hot water to a pan.

Bake until the center is set and top appears. Bake it for around 40 minutes. Switch off oven; partially open the screen. Give your cheesecake 30 minutes to cool down.

Remove the water pan and then remove foil. Loosen cheesecake sides with a knife; cool down for approx. 30 minutes on a wire rack. Refrigerate overnight and keep it covered.

You can top it with raspberries or anything you want!

23. Fruit Pizza

There is nothing better than a dessert that you can eat without any guilt, particularly when it is surmounted with delicious, colorful fruit. It requires 25 minutes for preparation and extra time for cooling. Then, you need 10 minutes for baking and more extra time for cooling.

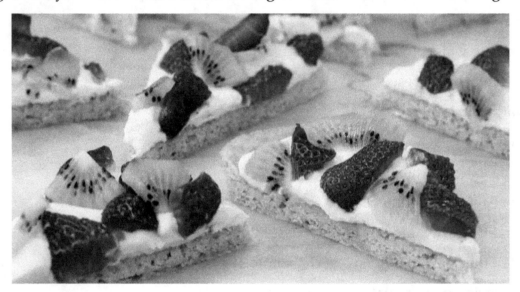

- All-purpose flour; 1 cup
- Butter; Half cup
- Confectioner sugar; ¼ cup

To prepare the glaze for your fruit pizza, you need the following ingredients.

- Cornstarch; 5 teaspoons
- Pineapple juice (unsweetened); 1 ¼ cups
- Lemon juice; 1 teaspoon

For the preparation of your fruit pizza topping, you require the following ingredients.

- Cream cheese (fat-free or low-fat); 8 oz.

- Sugar; 1/3 cup

- Vanilla extract; 1 teaspoon

- Fresh strawberries; 2 cups

- Fresh blueberries; 1 cup

- Oranges; 1 can

You can add more fruit if you like!

Preheat the oven to 350°. In a bowl, mix confectioners' sugar and flour; add butter until you get a crumbly texture. Press it in an ungreased pizza pan (12 inches). Bake until it gets light brown, for about 10 to 12 minutes. Cool it completely.

In a saucepan, mix glaze ingredients and keep mixing until it gets smooth. Then bring the mixture to a boil. Cook it until thick for approx. 2 minutes. Cool it.

Take a bowl, beat sugar, vanilla, and cream cheese until smooth. Now, spread it over the crust. You can top it with berries or mandarin oranges. And drizzle it with glaze. Keep it refrigerated until its cold and firm.

24. Chocolate Chip and Banana Cookies

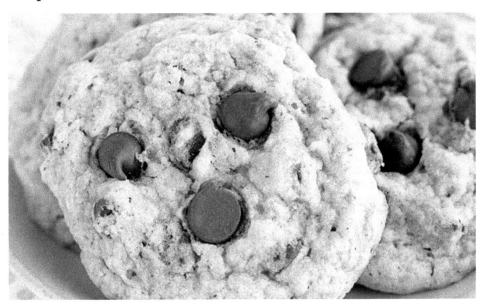

Such fluffy cookies with banana have a cakelike feel and plenty of taste that everybody seems to enjoy. You need 20 minutes for the preparation and then, baking requires 15 to 20 minutes. You can make more than 2 dozen cookies with the following ingredients.

- All-purpose flour; 1 ¼ cup

- Softened butter; 1/3 cup

- Large egg (1)

- Ripe banana (mashed); Half cup

- Vanilla extract; Half teaspoon

- Baking powder; 1 teaspoon

- Salt; ¼ teaspoon

- Baking soda; 1/8 teaspoon

- Chocolate chips (semisweet); 1 cup

In a bowl, mix butter and sugar until it gets fluffy. Beat in the egg, banana, and vanilla. Mix the flour with baking powder, salt, and baking soda; slowly add to the creamed mixture and mix it well. Then, stir in chocolate chips.

Drop the batter by tablespoonfuls with a distance of approx. 2 inches in between them on the baking sheets that you sprayed with cooking spray. Now, bake them at 350°; 13 to 16 minutes or wait until they are light brown. Cool them down on wire racks.

Tips:

Stir 1/2 cup of diced toasted walnuts or pecans into the batter for additional flavor. Toast almonds, bake for 5 to 10 minutes in a pan at 350 ° in an oven, or roast over low heat in a skillet until well browned.

Use ripe ones to produce the maximum taste when baking with bananas. Layer bananas

and an egg, mango, tomato or peach in a brown paper bag and leave it on your counter if you can spare a day or two. It will collect the fruit's ethylene gas, and speed the maturing cycle. To ripen bananas much quicker, place them on a baking sheet in their peels, and steam them up for 15 to 20 minutes in a 250° oven.

25. Strawberry Cheesecake – Choco-topped

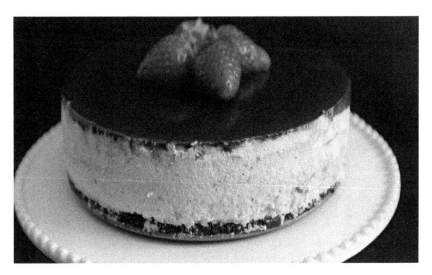

Creamy and soft, this beautiful dessert is something perfect for a summer party. It takes 35 minutes for preparation and then extra time for cooling. Another 10 minutes for baking and extra time for cooling it again. You can get 12 servings per cake.

- Crumbs – Graham Crackers; 1 ¼ cups
- Melted butter; ¼ cup
- Unflavored Gelatin; 2 envelopes
- Coldwater; Half cup
- Frozen Strawberries (unsweetened); 16 oz.
- Cream cheese (fat-free); 8 oz. 2 packets
- Cottage cheese (fat-free); 1 cup
- Sugar substitute; ¾ cup
- Whipped topping (low-fat); 8 oz.
- Topping (ice cream) chocolate; Half cup
- Fresh strawberries; 1 cup

Preheat the oven to 350°.

Mix the butter and crumbs; press downwards and 1-inch upwards in a 9 inches pan sprayed with cooking mist. Place on a sheet to bake. Bake for about 10 minutes, until set. Cool down on a wire rack.

Sprinkle gelatin in cold water in a small saucepan and then allow it to stand for 1 minute. Heat over low pressure, stir until the gelatin is dissolved completely; remove from fire.

Where appropriate, hull strawberries in a food processor. Empty it in a bowl. Then in a food processor, add cream cheese, cottage cheese, and substitute sugar, process it until it gets creamy and smooth. Gradually add gelatin mixture while it is being processed. Pureed strawberries are added; blend it well. Pass to a bowl; fold overtopping in 2 cups. Spread it on the crust. Cover, refrigerate for 2 to 3 hours.

Loosen the sides of the cheesecake using a knife and then remove the rim. You can use chocolate topping when serving or strawberries or whipped topping.

26. Cloud Bread

Try the Cloud Bread the next time you're having a pizza or some other meal containing slices of bread. Cloud Bread is a fully gluten-free option to low-carb, low-calorie, and low-fat food. It's a healthy choice and tastes good! You can also make pizza on a cloud bread!

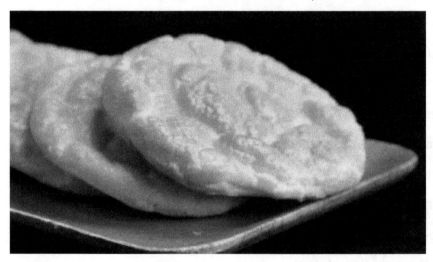

- Eggs (3)
- Softened cream cheese; 3 tablespoons
- Sugar; 1 teaspoon
- Cream of tartar; ¼ teaspoon

Preheat the oven to 300 degrees F. Then, coat 2 baking sheets using cooking spray.

In a bowl, mix cream cheese, sugar and egg yolks until smooth.

In another bowl, combine egg whites with tartar cream; beat with a high-speed electric mixer until fluffy and steep peaks shape. Gently fold the egg yolk mixture into a blend of egg white until well-integrated. Spoon mixture on baking sheets into 10 rounds.

Bake it for 25 to 30 minutes approx., or until it is golden brown. Let it cool for 5 minutes and then transfer it to a wire rack allowing it to cool completely.

Tips:

How to Store Cloud Bread: An airtight container is the best option if you want to store this bread.

How to Freeze Cloud Bread: Freeze after allowing it to cool. Remember that after being frozen the bread takes on a lighter texture.

What to Eat with Cloud Bread: This bread is a replacement for your regular bread. You can either eat it just like that or you can eat it with any spread. You can also make a sandwich using this bread. You can also make a pizza with this bread.

27. Peanut Butter Balls – No-Bake

Such peanut butter oatmeal balls are great for road trips and do not stick to your hands. They make a good snack! It takes only 10 minutes to prepare!

- Peanut Butter (chunky); 1/3 cup
- Honey; ¼ cup
- Vanilla extract; Half teaspoon
- Milk powder; 1/3 cup (fat-free)
- Oats (quick-cooking); 1/3 cup
- Crumbs; Graham Crackers; 2 tablespoons

Mix the honey and vanilla with peanut butter in a bowl. Stir in the oats, graham cracker crumbs, and the milk powder. Shape the mixture into small 1-inch balls. Now, cover and refrigerate before serving.

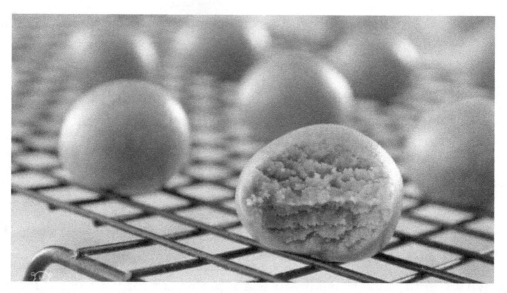

28. Orange Food Cake

Thanks to a touch of orange flavor swirled through every slice, a simple angel food cake is a heavenly indulgence. The preparation for this cake requires about 25 minutes and 30 minutes for baking. You can get 16 servings per cake.

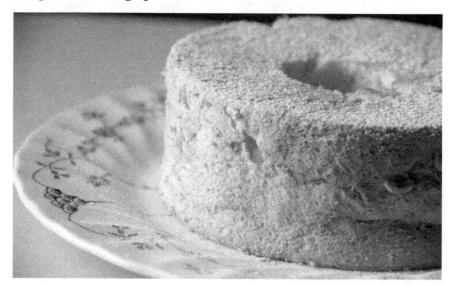

- Egg whites; 12 eggs
- All-purpose flour; 1 cup
- Sugar; 1 ¾ cup

- Cream of tartar; 1 ½ teaspoon

- Salt; Half teaspoon

- Almond extract; 1 teaspoon

- Vanilla extract; 1 teaspoon

- Orange zest (grated); 1 teaspoon

- Orange extract; 1 teaspoon

- Food color (red); 6 drops

- Food color (yellow); 6 drops

Put egg whites in a bowl; allow it to stand at room temperature for about 30 minutes. Mix flour and sugar together twice and then set it aside.

To egg whites, add salt, cream of tartar, and vanilla and almond extracts; beat at medium

speed until soft peaks develop. Then, add remaining sugar, around 2 teaspoons at a time, beating fast to create sharp, shiny peaks and dissolve sugar. Then, add in flour mixture, one and a half cup at a time.

Gently pour half of the batter into a 10 inches ungreased pan. Stir in the orange extract, orange zest, and the food color if necessary, to the remaining batter. Spoon orange batter gently over white batter. Cut with a knife into all sides to shake the orange and draw out the air pockets.

Bake at 375° for about 30 to 35 minutes on the oven's lowest rack. Bake it until it is light brown and its top appears to be dry. Then invert pan quickly and cool it for almost one

hour.

Remove the cake using a knife to loosen the sides and put it on a serving plate!

29. Meringue Cookies – Vanilla

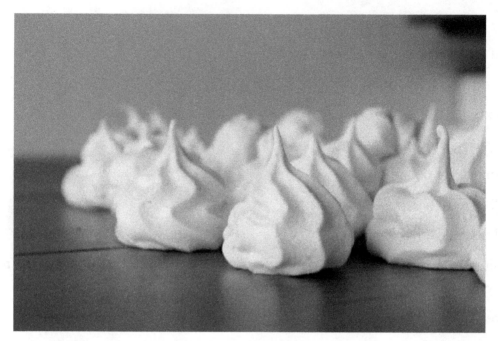

This cookie is sweet, airy and the ultimate fat-free dessert to help fight a desire for sweets. Ingredient preparation requires 20 minutes, and baking and standing require 40 minutes.

You can make approx. 5 dozen cookies with these ingredients.

- Egg whites (large); 3 eggs
- Vanilla extract; 1 ½ teaspoon
- Cream of tartar; ¼ teaspoon
- Sugar; 2/3 cup
- Dash salt

Pour egg whites in a bowl and allow them to stand for 30 minutes at room temperature. Preheat the oven to 250°. Then, add cream of tartar, salt, and vanilla to the egg whites and

beat the mixture until it gives a foam-like texture. Then, slowly add sugar and keep beating it high after each tablespoon is added until all the sugar dissolves. Keep beating it until it takes the form for approx. 7 minutes.

Cut a small hole in a pastry bag tip then insert a # 32-star tip. Fill the piping bag with your meringue mixture. Make cookie shapes using the tip on your piping bag, keep them small in size and at a distance from each other on the paper-lined baking sheets.

Bake for 40 to 45 minutes. Turn the oven off; keep the meringues in the oven for 1 hour and keep the oven door close. Clear from the oven; refrigerate fully on baking sheets. Cut the meringues from paper; place them at room temperature in an airtight container.

Tips:

- Room-temperature and old eggs make better meringues.

- On a dry day, it is better to make these cookies because on rainy or humid days they absorb moisture easily and become sticky.

30. Applesauce Brownies

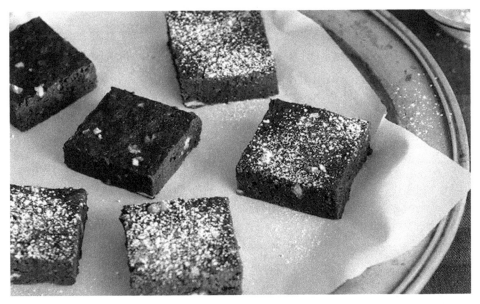

These brownies are easy to make and they taste good too. The preparation time for these brownie ingredients is 15 minutes approximately. Baking requires around 25 minutes along with cooling the brownies.

- Softened Butter; ¼ cup

- Sugar; ¾ cup

- Large egg

- All-purpose flour; 1 cup

- Baking cocoa; 1 tablespoon

- Baking soda; Half teaspoon

- Ground cinnamon; Half teaspoon

- Applesauce; 1 cup

For the topping, you need:

- Chocolate chips; Half cup

- Pecans or walnuts (chopped); Half cup

- Sugar; 1 tablespoon

Mix sugar and butter in a bowl. Beat an egg in. Then, mix the flour with cocoa, cinnamon, and baking soda. Then slowly add it to the creamy mixture and mix it well. Add in applesauce. Drop into an 8 inches baking pan (square) sprayed with cooking spray.

Combine the topping ingredients and sprinkle it over batter. Bake your brownies at 350° for about 25 minutes or keep check until the toothpick in the center comes out neat. Let it cool and then cut it in squares!

31. Oatmeal Cookies

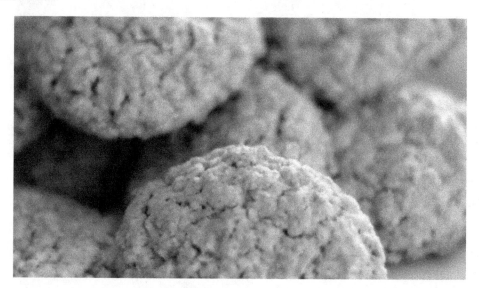

You need 35 to 40 minutes for preparation. Baking requires around 10 minutes per batch. You can make up to 5 dozen oatmeal cookies with the following ingredients.

- Hot water; 2 tablespoons

- Ground flaxseed; 1 tablespoon

- Dried chopped plums; 1 cup

- Dates (chopped); 1 cup

- Raisins; Half cup

- Softened butter; 1/3 cup

- Brown sugar; ¾ cup

- Large egg

- Vanilla extract; 2 teaspoons

- Applesauce (unsweetened); Half cup

- Maple syrup; ¼ cup

- Orange zest; 1 tablespoon

- Oats (quick-cooking); 3 cups

- All-purpose flour; 1 cup

- Whole-wheat flour; Half cup

- Baking soda; 1 teaspoon

- Ground cinnamon; 1 teaspoon

- Salt; Half teaspoon

- Ground nutmeg; ¼ teaspoon

- Ground cloves; ¼ teaspoon

Combine water and the flaxseed in a bowl. Combine the raisins, dates, and plums into another bowl. Cover with hot water. Let mixtures of flaxseed and plum stand for 10 minutes.

Then, mix butter and brown sugar in a bowl until it gets fluffy. Beat in Vanilla and Egg. Beat in applesauce, orange zest, and maple syrup. Combine the oats, flours, baking soda, salt, cinnamon, butter, cloves, and nutmeg; slowly apply and blend well to the creamed

mixture. Drain the mixture of the plum; add the mixture of the plum and the flaxseed to the flour.

Drop by teaspoonfuls 2 inches apart on a lightly greased baking sheet. Bake it at 350° for about 8 to 11 minutes. Let it cool for 2 minutes before you remove it from pans to the wire racks.

31. Peanut Butter Cake

The preparation time for this cake is 20 minutes. Baking requires 15 minutes along with cooling.

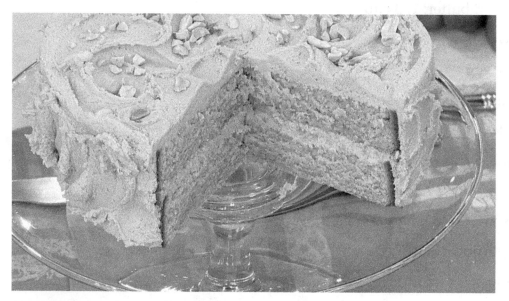

- Cubed butter; 6 tablespoons
- Peanut butter (creamy); Half cup
- Water; 1 cup
- All-purpose flour; 2 cups
- Sugar; 1 ½ cups
- Buttermilk; Half cup
- Applesauce (unsweetened); ¼ cup
- Large eggs (2); slightly beaten
- Baking powder; 1 ¼ teaspoon
- Vanilla extract; 1 teaspoon
- Salt; Half teaspoon

- Baking soda; ¼ teaspoon

For the cake's frosting, you need the following ingredients.

- Cubed butter; ¼ cup

- Peanut butter (creamy); ¼ cup

- Milk (fat-free); 2 tablespoons

- Confectioner sugar; 1 ¾ cup

- Vanilla extract; 1 teaspoon

Mix butter, water, and peanut butter in a saucepan and bring it to a boil. Remove it from heat immediately. Add flour, applesauce, sugar, eggs, buttermilk, salt, vanilla, baking soda, and baking powder. Mix it well.

Pour the mixture into a 15 by 10 by 1-inch baking pan covered with cooking spray. Bake it at 375° for about 15 to 20 minutes or wait until it is golden brown. Cool it for 20 to 30 minutes on a wire rack.

In a saucepan, mix peanut butter and butter on medium heat and then add milk. Boil it and then remove it from heat. Slowly add in vanilla and confectioner sugar and mix it well until it gets smooth. Spread it over a warm cake. Allow it to cool and then you can refrigerate the leftovers.

You can add nuts too!

32. Zucchini Bread – Diabetic

This bread is good and healthy for diabetes patients. It is low in sugar and low in carbs. And it is going to keep you healthy as well.

You need:

- Egg white; ¾ cup

- Applesauce (unsweetened); Half cup

- Melted butter (fat-free); Half cup

- Shredded Zucchini; 2 cups

- Shredded Carrot; Half cup

- Brown sugar; 6 tablespoons

- Baking powder; 1 teaspoon

- Baking soda; 1 teaspoon

- Cinnamon; 1 teaspoon

- Nutmeg; 1 teaspoon

- Salt; Half teaspoon

- Vanilla extract; 2 teaspoons

- Chopped walnuts; ¼ cup

- Whole-wheat flour; 2 cups

Preheat the oven to 350 degrees.

Then, grease and then flour two medium pans for loaves.

In a bowl combine brown sugar, egg, sugar, margarine, and apple sauce.

Then, add baking powder, cinnamon, baking soda, salt, nutmeg, and vanilla.

Then, add flour slowly and add shredded zucchini, nuts, and carrots.

Use a mixer or your hands to beat the mixture and pour the mixture into the loaf pans.

Bake it for 45 minutes. After that, let it cool.

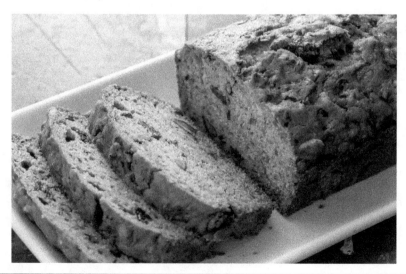

33. Berry Parfait

The perfect period for this parfait is mid-summer, as the northern forests are dense with blueberries. The total time required for this parfait is around 15 to 20 minutes which includes preparation as well.

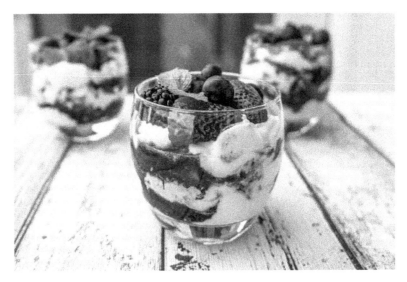

- Fresh strawberries; 2 cups; cut in half

- Fresh blueberries; 2 cups

- Walnut raspberry vinaigrette; 4 teaspoons

- Greek yogurt (strawberry or vanilla) fat-free; ¾ cup

- Fresh mint (minced); 2 teaspoons

- Shredded coconut (unsweetened); Optional

Put the blueberries and strawberries in separate cups. Drizzle Vinaigrette (2 teaspoons) on both the berries. Blend mint and yogurt in a bowl.

Place strawberries into four cups for the parfait. Cover each with blueberries and yogurt mixture. You can top it with shredded coconut as well if you want to!

34. Cinnamon Bars

In this recipe, the Classic bar follows good-for-you ingredients. If you can then keep them in a tin for a day after the bars are prepared. The next day, I think they taste much better. You can easily make around 2 dozen bars using the following ingredients. However, the total time required for the ingredient preparation is 20 to 25 minutes and 15 to 20 minutes for baking along with cooling.

- Whole wheat flour; Half cup

- All-purpose flour; Half cup

- Sugar; Half cup

- Ground cinnamon; 1 ½ teaspoon

- Baking powder; 1 ¼ teaspoon

- Baking soda; ¼ teaspoon

- Large egg; beaten

- Canola oil; 1/3 cup

- Applesauce (unsweetened); ¼ cup

- Honey; ¼ cup

- Walnuts (chopped); 1 cup

  Now, for the icing, you need the following ingredients.

- Melted butter; 2 tablespoons

- Water; 1 tablespoon

- Honey; 2 tablespoons

- Vanilla extract; 1 teaspoon

- Confectioner sugar; 1 cup

Preheat the oven to 350°. In a bowl, mix flours, baking powder, sugar, baking soda, and cinnamon. Mix oil, egg, honey, and applesauce in a bowl. Put it into the dry ingredients as it gets creamy and then add in walnuts.

Spread the batter into a 13 by 9 inches baking pan greased with cooking spray. Bake for about 15 to 20 minutes. You will know when it is done!

Now, combine your icing ingredients and spread it over the warm bars. Let the bars cool down entirely before you cut them!

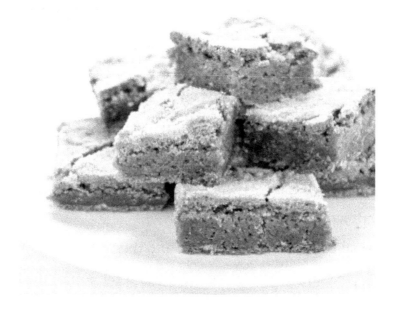

35. Banana Bread

It is a good snack for people with diabetes or prediabetic persons. Preparation time is about 10 to 15 minutes and baking requires almost 1 hour.

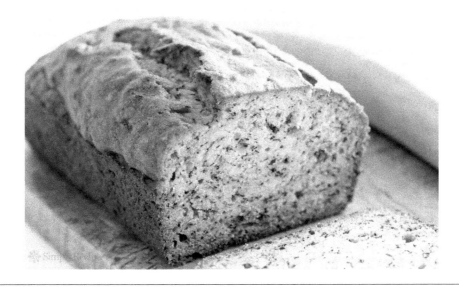

- Bananas (large); 2

- 2 Eggs

- Rapeseed oil; 4 tablespoons

- Vanilla extract; 1 teaspoon

- Brown sugar; 100 grams

- Flour (whole meal); 150 grams

- Baking powder; 2 teaspoons

- Mixed spice; 1 teaspoon (heaped)

- Walnuts (chopped); 50 grams

Preheat your oven to 170°C. Mash your bananas and once done, add eggs and then mix it well. Then add the vanilla extract, sugar, and oil. Mix it well.

Add in the flour, mixed spice, and baking powder and then add the chopped walnuts.

Pour the batter into a 2 pounds loaf tin, place the nuts on the top of the loaf, and bake it for 50 to 55 minutes, until a toothpick inserted into its center comes out neat.

Let it cool for 10 minutes in the pan and then you can remove it for it to cool down completely.

Tips:

You can also add other spices to it such as ground cinnamon or ground ginger, or you can use almonds instead of walnuts.

Freezing tips: You can freeze its slices in foil once it is prepared!

36.Chunky Apple Cake

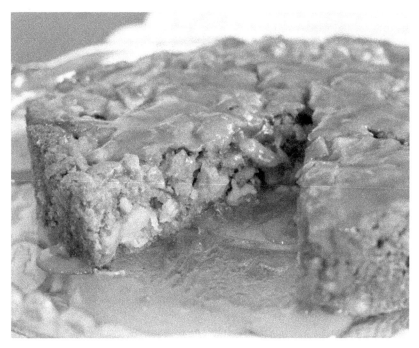

The preparation time for the ingredients required for this cake is approx. 30 minutes and 20 to 25 minutes for baking along with cooling. You can make 20 servings with the following ingredients.

- Large eggs; 2

- Brown sugar; Half cup

- Melted butter; 6 tablespoons

- Sugar; ¼ cup

- Vanilla extract; 2 teaspoons

- All-purpose flour; 2 cups

- Ground cinnamon; 2 teaspoons

- Baking powder; 1 teaspoon

- Baking soda; 1 teaspoon

- Salt; ¼ teaspoon

- Apples (shredded); 4; medium-sized

- Pecans (chopped); ¾ cup

Preheat your oven to 350 ° C. Coat a baking pan with cooking spray, 13 by 9 inches. Beat eggs, brown sugar, melted butter, sugar, and vanilla in a large bowl, until well mixed. Whisk sugar, flour, baking soda, salt, and baking powder in another bowl; slowly beat into a mixture of eggs. Stir in pecans and apples.

Switch to a prepared pan. Bake for 25-30 minutes or until the inserted toothpick in the center comes out of the cake clean. Cool on a wire rack, in the pan.

37. Elephant Ear Cookies

Now, this is something even your children will love to eat as a snack.

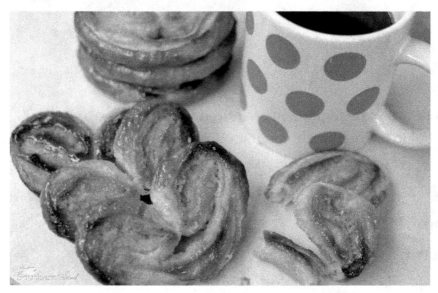

You need 35 to 40 minutes for the preparation and 10 to 15 minutes for baking these marvelous cookies. You can make approx. 2 dozen biscuits with the following ingredients.

- Active yeast (dry); ¼ oz.

- Warm water; ¼ cup

- All-purpose flour; 2 cups

- Sugar; 4 and a half teaspoons

- Salt; Half teaspoon

- Cubed butter (cold); 1/3 cup

- Milk (fat-free or low-fat); 1/3 cup

- Egg yolk (large egg)

For the filling, you need the following ingredients.

- Softened butter; 2 tablespoons

- Sugar; Half cup

- Ground cinnamon; 2 teaspoons

How to make cinnamon sugar? Here are the ingredients that you need to mix!

- Ground cinnamon; ¾ teaspoon

- Sugar; Half cup

Dissolve yeast in a ¼ cup warm. Mix the flour, salt, and sugar in a bowl; break into butter until you can see the crumbly texture. Stir in the yeast mixture the egg yolk and milk; add to the flour mixture, stir it to form the dough (your dough is going to be sticky). Cover it with plastic wrap. Then, cool down for 2 hours approx.

Preheat the oven until 375 ° C. Turn the dough on a floured wooden mat; roll the dough into a rectangle of 18 by 10 inches. Layer to about 1/4 inches with melted butter. For rims. Mix cinnamon and sugar; scatter on milk. Roll up type jelly-roll, starting with its long side; pinch the seam to close. Cut into 24 parts, crosswise. Cover slices with plastic wrap up to flattening level.

In a bowl, mix the cinnamon sugar ingredients. Place a strip of waxed paper 6 inches square on a working surface; sprinkle it with cinnamon sugar. Then, top it with one piece of dough; add cinnamon sugar (half teaspoon) to sprinkle on the dough. Roll the dough down to a diameter of 4 inches. Flip the dough onto a baking sheet lined with the cooking spray using waxed paper. Repeat the steps with the remaining ingredients, separating the slices by 2 inches. Bake for 7 to 9 minutes or to brown until golden. Cool on rack wire.

38.Masala Bread Rolls – Whole Wheat

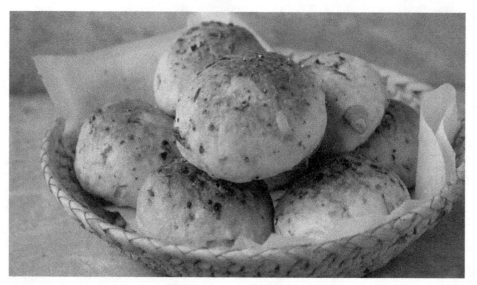

For these delicious bread rolls, different steps require different time. Preparation is done in approx. 10 to 15 minutes. Cooking requires about 2 to 5 minutes and 25 to 35 minutes for baking. You can make Nine bread rolls using the following ingredients.

- Whole wheat flour; 2 cups

- Instant yeast; 2 teaspoons

- Sugar; Half teaspoon

- Butter (low-fat); 2 teaspoons

- Salt for taste

- Melted butter (low fat) for brushing; ¼ teaspoon

To prepare the masala for the bread rolls, you need the following ingredients.

- Oil; 1 teaspoon

- Onions (chopped); ¼ cup

- Garlic (chopped); 1 tablespoon

- Green chilies (chopped); a Half tablespoon

- Chopped cilantro; ½ cup

- Turmeric powder; ¼ teaspoon

- Salt for taste

To prepare the masala:

Heat the oil or low-fat butter in a pan. If it is a non-stick pan, then it is better. Then, add onions, green chilies, and garlic in the pan. Cook it for 1 minute on medium flame.

Then, add cilantro, turmeric, salt, and chili powder. Mix it properly. Then cook it for 1 minute on a medium flame.

Put it aside to cool it down and your masala is ready.

To prepare the Bread Rolls:

In a shallow pot, mix the yeast with warm water, cover it with a lid and leave it aside for ten minutes. Now, in a deep tub, add the whole wheat flour, salt, butter, and the yeast mixture and knead it into a gentle dough with warm water.

Cover with a moist muslin cloth over the dough and held aside for 20 minutes or until the dough rises a bit.

Now apply the masala powdered, and knead properly.

Divide the dough into 9 equal parts and roll each part into a disk, then put the dough on the grated baking tray.

Then, over them with a moist cloth of muslin and keep them in a warm spot for around 30 minutes or until they grow up.

Bake them in a preheated oven for 20 to 25 minutes, at 200 degrees. Brush the melted butter to the bread rolls and serve them!

39.Oatmeal Bread – Gingerbread

The preparation time for this bread is 10 minutes and approx. 3 hours for baking! You can easily make 1 loaf using the following ingredients.

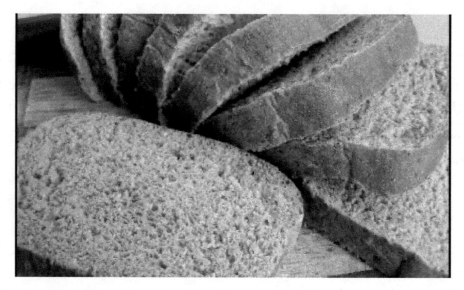

- Water; 1 cup + 1 tablespoon

- Molasses; Half cup

- Canola oil; 1 tablespoon

- Bread flour; 3 cups

- Oats; 1 cup

- Ground cinnamon; 1 and a half teaspoon

- Ground ginger; 1 teaspoon or Half more

- Salt; 1 teaspoon

- Orange zest (grated); Half teaspoon

- Ground nutmeg; ¼ teaspoon

- Ground cloves; ¼ teaspoon

- Active yeast; ¼ oz.

Layer all ingredients in the bread machine pan in the order suggested by the maker. Pick a simple environment for the bread. Pick the color of the crust and size of the loaf, if appropriate.

Bake according to the instructions of the bread machine (check the dough after five minutes of mixing; apply 1 to 2 spoons of water or flour if necessary).

40.Light Chocolate Pudding

This pudding is creamy and it is light just as promised! You need 10 minutes for preparation and 15 to 20 minutes for cooking it along with cooling. You can make 4 servings out of the following ingredients.

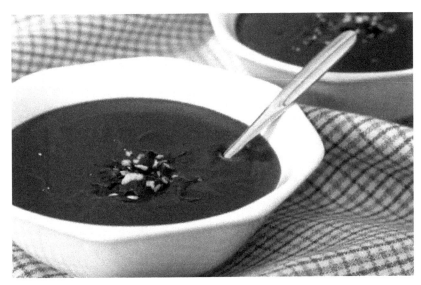

- Cornstarch; 3 tablespoons
- Sugar; 2 tablespoons
- Baking cocoa; 2 tablespoons
- Salt; 1/8 teaspoon
- Soy milk (chocolate); 2 cups
- Vanilla extract; 1 teaspoon

Add the cornstarch, cocoa, sugar, salt in a hot, heavy saucepan. Whisk in some milk. Cook and mix over medium heat until bubbly and thickened. Reduce heat to low; boil and stir for 2 minutes.

Remove the saucepan from heat and then stir vanilla in. Cool for 15 minutes.

Transfer to plates for dessert. Cover, refrigerate, for 30 minutes, or until cold.

41. Lemon Cheese Bars

These delicious bars take 15 to 20 minutes for preparation along with 25 to 30 minutes for baking and more time for cooling. You can prepare 2 dozen bars with the following ingredients.

- Lemon cake mix; 1 packet

- Egg substitute; Half cup

- Canola oil; 1/3 cup

- Cream cheese (low-fat); 8 oz.

- Sugar; 1/3 cup

- Lemon juice; 1 teaspoon

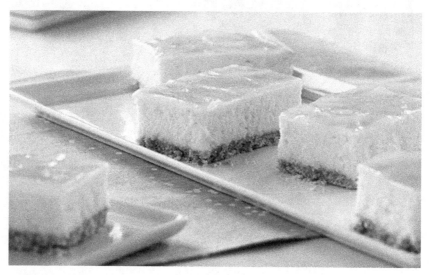

Preheat your oven to 350 ° C. Combine cake mix, the egg substitute, and oil in a deep bowl; combine until smooth. To top off-reserve 1/2 cup mixture. Place the excess mixture into the bottom of a baking sheet with cooking spray lined with 13 by 9 inches. Bake for 11-13 minutes or until light brown around the bottom.

Mix cream cheese, sugar, and lemon juice in a medium cup, until smooth. Add the remaining egg substitute; beat only until blended at a low level. Disseminate over salt. Crumble is reserved for filling over top.

Bake for 11-13 minutes, or until it is ready to complete. Cooldown 1 hour on a wire rack. Split these into plates. Keep the leftover in your refrigerator.

42. Almond Hazelnut Biscotti

You need 30 minutes for preparation and 30 minutes for baking. You can make approx. 2 dozen biscotti using the following ingredients.

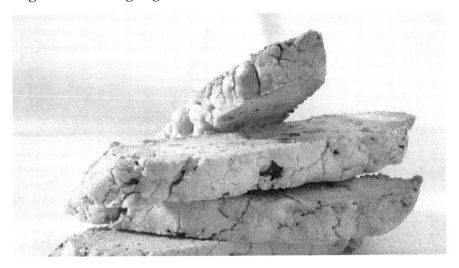

- Large eggs; 2
- Sugar; ¾ cup
- Vanilla extract; 2 teaspoons
- Almond extract; ¾ teaspoon
- All-purpose flour; 1 2/3 cup
- Salt; ¼ teaspoon
- Baking soda; Half teaspoon
- Hazelnuts (chopped and toasted); 2/3 cup
- Almonds (sliced and toasted); ¼ cup

Toast almonds, bake for 5-10 minutes in a shallow pan in a 350 ° oven, or roast over low heat in a skillet until well browned and stirring regularly.

Preheat your oven to 350 ° C. Beat eggs, sugar, and spices in a bowl, until well combined. Whisk the rice, baking soda and salt together in another bowl; slowly whisk in the egg mixture. Stir in the nuts (the mixture becomes stiff).

Divide the batter into two. Using lightly floured palms, form each section on a parchment-lined baking sheet into a rectangle measuring 9 by 2 inches. Bake for about 20 minutes, until golden brown.

Cool on wire racks till firm on pans. Reduce the level on the oven to 325 °. Move rectangles boiled to a cutting plate. Cut diagonally through 3/4-in, use a serrated knife. Sliced slices. Put them on baking sheets, cut the side down.

Bake for 5-7 minutes per leg, until lightly browned. Remove to wire racks from the pans; cool down completely. Store in a container that is airtight.

43. Banana Cereal Popsicles

15 minutes for preparation and almost 1 hour for freezing. Make 8 pops with the following ingredients.

- Strawberry yogurt; ¾ cup
- Bananas (medium-sized) cut in half; 4
- Cereal; Fruity Pebbles; 2 cups
- Wooden sticks; 8

Put yogurt and cereal in individual, shallow bowls. Attach pop sticks to the banana from the side that you cut. Dip the bananas in yogurt, then roll them to cover in cereal. Switch to waxed baking sheets lined with parchment.

Freeze up for around 1 hour, before solid. Transfer to containers with airtight freezer; seal containers, and return pops to the freezer.

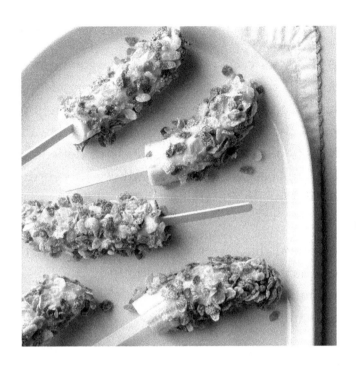

Tips:

• Switch it to vanilla yogurt or Cocoa Pebbles.

• This basic formula accounts for the use of mature and sweet but yet strong bananas. Search for bananas with little to no green, with no gray or black stains on them. This is a clever way of utilizing a load of extra bananas.

Conclusion

A low-carb diet can help diabetics control their blood sugar rates easier. Carbohydrates are more likely to boost blood glucose than other products, suggesting the body will generate more insulin to absorb them. Reducing the intake of carb may help to stabilize blood glucose. It can also counteract some of the other diabetes effects, such as heart diseases or weight gain. More than that, low-carb diets often bear other hazards of deficits in vitamins and minerals. Low carb diets are difficult for certain people to adhere to overtime. People should try to speak to a doctor before making major dietary adjustments, especially those that involve diabetes control.

While the link among sugar and diabetes remains uncertain, a reduction in the diet's added sugar and refined food may help an individual avoid type 2 diabetes. Other adjustments to the lifestyle can help decrease the risk of type 2 diabetes or assist people with diabetes to deal with their problems and avoid complications.

A low-carb diet may help diabetes sufferers prevent complications. This will help maintain the blood pressure down, rising energy slumps, support weight reduction, and even change the disease path. A low-carb diet can be the first line of therapy for patients who choose to delay drugs, or whose doctor has just newly identified diabetes. Low-carb diets are not an unhealthy low-carb diet for everyone — like living off fried, fatty meats — might be even more harmful to a person's health than lots of carbs.

Similarly, a person must be able to stick to a long-term low-carb diet to fully reap its benefits. Please speak to a specialist or dietitian before carrying out some new diet. People may consider keeping a list of their symptoms and what they've consumed, to assess how the diet affects their long-time wellbeing.

Renal Diet Cookbook

The Easy-to-Follow Beginners Guide for The Best 48 Low Sodium and Low Potassium Recipes recommended to Manage and Avoid Kidney Disease and Live a Healthy Life without Dialysis

By

Oliver Gundry

Introduction

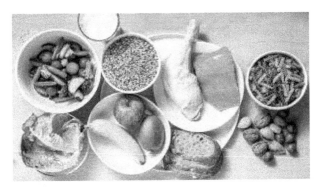

Chronic kidney disease, affects over thirty million Americans. Only a small fraction of those diagnosed will ever have to face a kidney transplant or dialysis. For more the fifty years, people have known that diet has a large impact on the outcome of CKD patients by slowing the rate of their progression, delaying the onset of their symptoms, decreasing the risk of cardiovascular problems, and improving the internal environment of their body. For those who already suffer from cardiovascular disease, high blood pressure, high cholesterol, or diabetes, dietary changes can go a long way to help stabilize the function of the kidneys and improve survival.

Unfortunately, for most newly diagnosed CKD patients, learning to follow the renal diet can be challenging. This can be even scarier if they have already been told to reduce their sugar intake or fats. The main question most people will have when facing a renal diet is "With all of these restrictions, what can I eat?" They are afraid that they will have to eat boring and bland foods, which makes any diet unsustainable and difficult to follow.

This book is here to help with just that. Managing CKD will require lifestyle changes, but you're not alone. But without knowing what can happen, fear, anxiety, depression, and uncertainty are common among CKD patients. A lot may even feel that dialysis is inevitable, and you could find yourself wondering it's worth your time and effort. Only one in fifty people diagnosed with CKD faces dialysis. With the right tools, you can delay and prevent end-stage renal disease and dialysis. With simple management strategies, you can live a full and productive life.

Chapter 1

What Is Kidney Disease

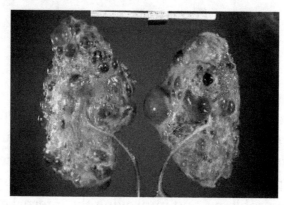

It is going to sound scary when you get diagnosed with chronic kidney disease and you probably have a lot of question. This disease can be managed very well. It will take some exploration, patience, and time to see the big picture. Your first step to managing kidney disease is being able to understand it. Let's take a look at the role your kidneys play in your health, how your diet plays an important role in helping to manage kidney disease, and what happens when you develop kidney disease.

Once you have been diagnosed with CKD, it will be helpful to explore this disease and learn about some normal symptoms. A simple definition is a gradual loss of the function of your kidneys. Because our bodies constantly produce waste, our kidneys play a big role to remove these toxins and keep our system working properly. Tests will be done to measure the level of waste in your blood and figure out how well your kidneys are working. Your doctor will be able to find out the filtration rate of your kidneys and figure out what stage of CKD you are in.

There are five stages that show how the kidneys function. Within the early stages, people won't experience any symptoms, and it is very easy to manage. Oftentimes, kidney disease isn't found until it becomes advanced. Most symptoms don't appear until the toxins build-up in the body from the damage that has been done to the kidneys. This usually happens in the later stages. Changes in how you urinate, vomiting, nausea, swelling, and itching could be caused by decreased ability to filtrate the toxins. This is why an early diagnosis that is critical to positive outcomes can come later when the disease has progressed.

There isn't a cure for CKD, but you can manage this disease. Making changes to your lifestyle and diet can slow down the progression and help you stay away from symptoms that normally start to show up later. These lifestyle changes can improve your total health and allow you to manage other conditions. Once you begin making changes to your daily food habits, you will see improvement in these conditions including diabetes and hypertension.

You can live a happy, healthy, and long life while managing CKD and making changes early can slow down the progression of this disease for years.

How the Kidneys Work

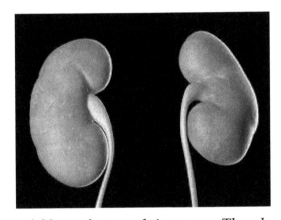

Our kidneys are bean-shaped filters that work in teams. They have a very important job since they keep our bodies stable. They use signals from the body like blood pressure and sodium content to help keep us hydrated and our blood pressure stable.

If the kidneys don't function right, there are numerous problems that could happen. When the filtration of these toxins becomes slow, these harmful chemicals can build up and cause other reactions within the body like vomiting, nausea, and rashes. When the kidney's functions continue to decrease, its ability to get rid of water and release hormones that control blood pressure can also be affected. Symptoms such as high blood pressure or retaining water in your feet might happen. With time having reduced kidney function could cause long-term health problems such as osteoporosis or anemia.

The kidneys work hard, so we have to protect them. They can filter around 120 to 150 quarts of blood each day. This will create between 1 and 2 quarts of urine that are made up of excess fluid and waste products.

Causes

Conditions like hypertension and diabetes have been associated with kidney disease and play key roles in decreasing how these organs function. Let's look at some common causes of CKD and what you need to think about if you have more than one of the following conditions.

Diabetes

This disease changes how your body uses and produces insulin. This hormone gets released from the pancreas that gets sugar from the blood and then sends it to other organs that need it to function properly. If you have been diagnosed with diabetes, there is a chance you know all these information already and you have learned how to manage it with medicine and diet.

If your diabetes is uncontrolled or chronic, it could damage your kidneys, and it is a major factor in developing CKD. Diabetes is the main cause of kidney disease. One of the jobs for kidneys is filtering the fluid in the body and getting rid of the waste along with water that isn't needed. Think about this fluid going through the kidneys constantly 24 hours a day. Normal filtration systems are strong enough to handle all the pressure. If there are large sugar molecules in the blood, this can increase the pressure that is put on the filter and, over time, it will break.

Hypertension/High Blood Pressure

This can cause kidney damage and could be caused by damage to the kidneys. The blood vessels send all the blood through the entire body. This alone puts pressure on the artery walls. If this pressure becomes too high, it might damage the vessel walls, especially the small vessels like the ones found inside the kidneys. The blood vessels that go through the kidneys change molecules during this filtration process. If these walls get damaged, it could hurt how the filtration process works and causes the kidneys to become damaged and, thus, causing CKD.

The kidney's main function is controlling blood pressure by producing hormones. When the kidneys get damaged, they won't be able to regulate these hormones, and your blood pressure could go up. If you struggle to control your hypertension or want to regulate your blood pressure, managing your lifestyle and diet could help. Many elements of a kidney- friendly diet can help manage your hypertension. It is important to think about this as you figure out what changes you want to make for the good of your health.

Treating Chronic Kidney Disease

Being able to manage chronic kidney disease takes a lot of lifestyle changes, dietary modifications, and working with your doctors. You can up your chances for better outcomes by learning about the disease and finding out everything you can about the choices you make. Knowledge is power, so grab everything you can. This is very true with you have chronic kidney disease.

Diet

Learning how to eat with CKD is a bit overwhelming, but with anything that is new, when you begin practicing it, it will soon be a normal part of your life that won't require any thought. The basic guideline is restricting phosphorus, potassium, sodium, protein, and at times, fluids. This is all based on the results of your blood work. Your health care professional and dietitian can make a diet plan specifically for your needs. The rest is totally up to you. How well you comply with restrictions on your diet has a large influence on how fast the disease progresses.

Lifestyle

Just like a diet, the choices you make in life plays a huge part in managing your CKD. Staying away from alcohol, quitting smoking, reducing stress, managing your weight, getting enough sleep, and exercising regularly are all great lifestyle practices. They could help you reduce or manage your risk of chronic diseases like high blood pressure, diabetes, and heart disease. Lifestyle choices that are practiced on a regular basis could make a large difference in the way you feel emotionally and physically.

Health Care Team

Managing and treating your chronic kidney disease needs to involve a good health care team. You should have a dietitian, social workers, nurses, and a renal doctor. These people all give specific expertise. When they work together, they are a professional support system to guide and educate you about your chronic kidney disease. Health care professionals who are experts in renal failure will give you the best information. Make sure they work together to create an individual plan for your specific needs. You have to be honest and open with your team about the way you feel and the diet and lifestyle choices you make for them to help you. They aren't going to judge you but help you make the right choices so you can manage your CKD.

Slowing Down Kidney Disease

Now that you know what CKD is, let's look at how to slow the progress. This information will give you specific steps to do to develop a healthier lifestyle and diet. You have to keep an open mind and take it one step at a time. Having a positive attitude is important and the way you embrace the steps will determine how you manage your kidney disease. With some determination and willpower from you, you will soon be in charge of your destiny and health.

1. Commit

You might begin feeling a bit overwhelmed when you think about this disease. Take a few deep breaths. Everything is going to be fine because you've got this. Just like any life changes, creating new habits will take time. Just take it one day at a time. Start preparing yourself mentally by telling yourself that you can control this disease by managing your lifestyle and diet.

Promise yourself that you will do your best every day to change your lifestyle and habits. Your commitment to yourself and your motivation to follow through will help you manage your kidney disease. Keep in mind that the earlier this disease gets detected, the better you can treat it. There is a goal for your treatment: slowing down the disease and keeping it from getting any worse. This is one good thing about kidney disease: It lets you take control so you can manage it.

2. Know Your Nutritional Needs

There isn't one diet plan that will be right for everybody who has kidney disease. What you are able to eat is going to change with time. It all depends on how well your kidneys function and factors such as being a diabetic. If you can work closely with your health team and constantly learning, you will be able to make healthy choices that will fit your needs. You can manage your disease and be successful.

Here are some basic guidelines that are useful for anyone who has chronic kidney disease:

Protein

Protein is found in plant and animal foods. Protein is a macronutrient that is needed for a healthy body. For people who have chronic kidney disease having too much isn't good. As the function of the kidney's decline, the body doesn't have the ability to get rid of the waste that gets produced when protein gets broken down and it begins to build up in the blood. The correct amount of protein depends on what stage your kidney disease is in, your body size, appetite, levels of albumin, and other factors. A dietitian could help you figure out your daily limits of protein intake. Here is a general guideline to give you an idea of the amount of protein you should be eating: 37 to 41 grams of protein daily.

If you have been diagnosed with CKD and you smoke, you are increasing the risk of developing end-stage renal disease. Smoking harms almost every organ in the body. Stopping might be the most important thing you can do for your body. Talk with your doctor about ways to help you stop.

Fats

When you are going through times where you are having to restrict what you eat, it is good to know that being able to eat healthy fats is another macronutrient that you need to include daily. Eating healthy fats makes sure you are getting all the essential fatty acids that can help your body in many ways. Polyunsaturated and monounsaturated fats are both unsaturated fats but they are healthy fats because of their benefits to the heart like decreasing LDL, increasing HDL, and lowering the total cholesterol levels. The correct types of fat might decrease inflammation within the body and will protect your kidney from more damage. You should try to include small amounts of these fats into your daily diet.

Carbohydrates

Carbs are another macronutrient that the body needs. This is what the body uses for energy. They also give the body many minerals, fiber, and vitamins that help protect the body. The body needs 130 grams of carbs daily for normal function.

Sodium

Consuming too much sodium makes you thirsty. This can cause increased blood pressure and swelling. Having high blood pressure could cause even more damage to the kidneys that are already unhealthy. Consuming less sodium will lower blood pressure and could slow down chronic kidney disease. The normal recommendation for anyone who has CKD is to keep their sodium intake around 2,000 mg daily. To have the best success is remembering that eating fresh is the best. Sodium can be found in all pickled, cured, salted, or processed foods. Fast foods, frozen and canned can also be high in sodium. Foods that are less processed will have the least amount of sodium. If going "fresh is the best" is the lifestyle change you want to do, you will be giving your body a healthy boost.

Potassium

Potassium can be found in many beverages and foods. It has an important role. It regulates the heartbeat and keeps muscles functioning. People who have kidneys that aren't healthy will need to limit their intake of foods that will increase how much potassium is in the blood. It might increase it to dangerous levels. Eating a diet that restricts your level of potassium means eating around 2.000 milligrams each day. Your dietitian or doctor can tell you what level of potassium would be right for you based on your individual needs and blood work.

In order to lessen the buildup of potassium, you have to know what foods are low and high in potassium. This way you know what foods to be careful around.

Phosphorus

Kidneys that are healthy can help the body regulate phosphorus. When you have CKD, your kidneys can't remove excess phosphorus or get rid of it. This results in high levels of phosphorus in the blood and causes the body to pull calcium from bones. This, in turn, will lead the brittle and weak bones. Having elevated levels of calcium and phosphorus could lead to dangerous mineral deposits in the soft tissues of the body. This is called calciphylaxis.

Phosphorus can be found naturally in plant and animal proteins and in larger levels in processed foods. By choosing foods that are low in phosphorus will keep the phosphorus levels in your body safe. The main rule to keep from eating unwanted phosphors goes back to "fresh is the best" concept. Basically stay away from all process foods. Normal phosphorus intake for anyone who has CKD needs to be around 800 to 1,000 milligrams daily.

Supplements and Vitamins

Instead of relying on supplements, you need to follow a balanced diet. This is the best way to get the number of vitamins your body needs each day. Because of the restrictive CKD diet, it can be hard to get the necessary nutrients and vitamins you need. Anyone who has CKD will have greater needs for vitamins that are water soluble. Certain renal supplements are needed to get the needed extra water soluble vitamins. Renal vitamins could be small doses of vitamin C, biotin, pantothenic acid, niacin, folic acid, Vitamins B12, B6, B2, and B1.

The kidney converts inactive vitamin D to an active vitamin D so our bodies can use it. With CKD, kidneys lose the ability to do this. Your health care provider could check your parathyroid hormone, phosphorus, and calcium levels to figure out if you need to take any supplements of active vitamin D. This type of vitamin D requires a prescription.

If your doctor hasn't prescribed a supplement, don't hesitate to ask them if you would benefit from one. To help keep you healthy, only use supplements that have been approved by your dietitian or doctor.

Fluids

A main function for the kidneys is regulating the balance of fluids in the body. For many individuals who have CKD, you don't have to restrict your fluid intake if your output is normal. As the disease progresses, there will be a decline in output and an increase in retention. If this happens, restricting fluids will become necessary. You have to pay attention to how much fluid you are releasing. Let your health care team know if you see that your output is declining. They will be able to tell you how much fluid you should limit on a daily basis to keep healthy fluid levels to prevent an overload of fluid in the body along with other complications that are associated with extra fluid buildup like congestive heart failure, pulmonary edema, edema, and high blood pressure.

3. Understand Your Calorie Requirements

Each person's calorie requirements will be different and it doesn't matter if they do or don't have CKD. If they do have CKD, picking the correct foods and eating the right amount of calories will help your body. Calories give us the energy to function daily. They can help to slow the progression of kidney disease, keep a healthy weight, avoid losing muscle mass, prevent infections. Eating too many calories could cause weight gain, and that can put more of a burden on your kidneys. It is important that you get the correct amount of calories. The amount of calories for a person with CKD is about 60 to 70 calories per pound of body weight. If you weigh about 150 pounds, you need to consume around 2,000 calories per day.

4. Read Food Labels

It takes time to learn the renal diet and make it a part of your life. Lucky for you all packaged foods come with nutrition labels along with an ingredient list. You need to read these labels so you can choose the right foods for your nutrition needs.
The main ingredients you need to look for on the labels are potassium, phosphorus, sodium, and fat. Manufacturers of food are required by law to list the sodium and fat content of the food. They aren't required to list potassium or phosphorus. It is important to find this information in other places like the internet or books.

5. Portion Control

When you have kidney disease, controlling your portions is important. This doesn't mean you have to starve yourself. It doesn't matter what stage of CKD you are in but eating moderately is important when preserving your kidney health. The biggest part is making sure you don't feel deprived. You can enjoy many different foods as long as they are kidney- friendly and don't overeat. When you cut back on foods that could harm your health and you are careful about what you eat, you are learning portion control. Make a habit of limiting specific foods and eating in moderation when following a kidney diet. It just takes having an informed game plan, resolve, and time.

Picking the correct foods is critical to your kidneys. They are counting on you to give them the correct nutrients so they can function their best. This included minerals, vitamins, fats, carbohydrates, and protein. Too much of any one could harm your body and make your kidneys work harder to get rid of the toxins.

One way to use portion control and picking the correct foods is practicing trying to balance your plate. See your plate with half of it vegetables, a quarter of its protein, and the other quarter carbohydrates.

There is quite a bit of information to learn and it is going to take some time to remember it. That is fine. Take some time and commit to learning. Before you know it, you will be an expert. You will know your body, what it needs in order to thrive and keep your kidneys in good health.

Chapter 2

Causes Of Kidney Disease

POLYCYSTIC KIDNEY DISEASE

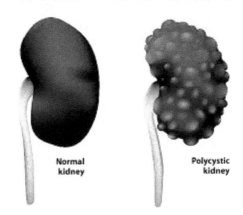

Normal kidney   Polycystic kidney

The major function of the kidney is to produce urine through the filtration of the excess water out of your blood. To ensure the proper functioning of our body, the kidneys maintain the level of electrolytes like potassium, calcium, sodium, and phosphorus. Also, your kidneys produce hormones that regulate blood pressure, produce red blood cells, and maintain the strength of your bones. Kidney disease progressively becomes worse and could result in kidney failure. If you are experiencing kidney failure, a kidney transplant or dialysis is required to keep you healthy. Early detection helps you to make the necessary adjustments to conserve your kidney functions.

How common is CKD?

In the United States, CKD is common in adults. The American adults that have CKD might be more than 30 million.

Conditions that Usually Lead to CKD

You have a greater chance of experiencing kidney disease if you have

Diabetes: The number one cause of CKD is diabetes. Diabetes is due to an increase in the levels of blood sugar or blood glucose that can then result in the damage of the blood vessels in your kidneys. Out of 3 adults with diabetes, it is likely that 1 person would suffer from CKD.

High blood pressure: The second highest cause of CKD is high blood pressure. High blood pressure, like diabetes, can cause damage in the blood vessels in your kidneys. Out of 5 adults with high blood pressure, 1 of them possibly has CKD.

Heart disease: Studies have discovered a connection between kidney and heart diseases. People that have heart disease have a greater chance of developing kidney disease and people with kidney disease have a greater chance of developing heart diseases. Scientists are carrying out extensive research to fully comprehend the relationship between heart disease and kidney disease.

Family history of kidney failure: You have a greater chance of developing CKD if your father, mother, brother or sister has kidney failure. If you have kidney disease, motivate your family to get tested. Discuss with your family on special family occasions using information from the family health reunion guide.

Note that the older you become, the higher your risk of developing kidney disease. You have a greater chance of developing kidney disease if you have had heart disease, diabetes, or high blood pressure for a long time. American Indians, Hispanics, and African Americans have a higher chance of developing CKD. The increased risk is primarily as a result of an increased rate of high blood pressure and diabetes in these people. Researchers are studying other probable causes for this higher risk.

Chapter 3

Renal Diet And Its Benefits

A renal diet is a diet that is meant to help people with a kidney disease. If you suffer from kidney diseases you will need to monitor and control several important nutrients. As such people with kidney diseases have to follow a specific diet that helps them meet those criteria and they all need to reduce certain things in their diet such as sodium potassium and phosphorus.

The reason that a kidney patient needs to monitor their sodium is because too much can be harmful. This is because their kidneys are already having trouble with the waste and they are unable to eliminate the extra fluid and sodium in the body. As they both begin to build-up in their tissues and in their bloodstream they could experience the following.

- High blood pressure
- Edema (this is in the hands, face and legs)
- Increased thirst
- Heart failure-because the extra fluid in the bloodstream can overwork your heart which makes it weak and enlarged.
- Shortness of breath because the excess causes build up in your lungs. This caused you to have a breaking issue.

They need to monitor potassium as well. Potassium helps make your heart beat regular and helps your muscles work the way they are supposed to. The kidneys help maintain the proper amount of potassium in your body and they expel the excess amount into your urine. When these organs no longer work right and they can't get rid of the excess, it builds up in your body. This results in a condition that is known as hyperkalemia and this condition is known for being able to give you the following issues.

- Weakness of the muscles
- Slow pulse
- Heart attacks
- Irregular heartbeat
- Death

Phosphorus is another mineral that is vital to the maintenance of your bones and development and its job is to assist the connective tissue and organs. However normal working kidneys can remove the excess in your blood but when your kidney function is compromised they no longer have the ability to do this. As such, the high levels can pull the calcium out of your bones which weakens them.

This also makes calcium deposits in the following areas of your body and brings them to an unsafe level:

Your eyes

- Your lungs
- Your blood vessels
- Your heart

Chapter 4

What To Eat And What To Avoid

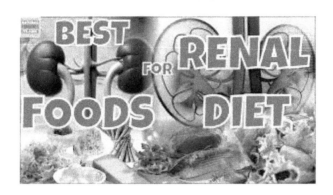

What to Avoid

Some Cereals

Oatmeal, whole wheat grains, cookies, pancakes, waffles, muffins, biscuits, pretzels.

Some Meats and Fish

Deli meats, salmon, sardines, organ meats.

Drinks to Avoid

Colas, soft drinks.

Avoid Foods High in Potassium:

Bananas, avocados, most fish, potatoes, spinach, artichokes, dates, oranges.

Avoid Foods High in Phosphorous

Processed cheese, red meat, fast food, milk, colas, canned fish.

Avoid Foods High in Sodium

Canned foods, processed foods, sauces, condiments, soy sauce, seasonings and salt added to your foods, avoid packaged or deli meats and control your portions well.

Limit Your Intake of The Following Foods:

Peanut butter, nuts in general, beans, seeds, butter or margarine.

What To Eat

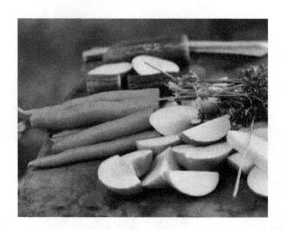

Drinks

You can favor the following drinks in your renal diet: some water, citrus based juices, wine, cranberry juice. Please consult with your doctor to know the right amount of fluids you should drink, depending on your kidneys conditions and the treatments you are going under. Don't forget to include the liquids included in soups or other liquid dishes.

Eat Plenty of Vegetables

Corn, carrot, cabbage peas, eggplants, celery, lettuce, asparagus, bean sprouts, red bell peppers, onions, garlic, cauliflower.

Choose Low Sugar Fruits

Cranberries, apples, cherries, blackberries, blueberries, mangoes, pears, peaches, grapes.
Others

Privilege olive oil to other oils, eggs, lean meats such poultry, beef, pork, coriander, ginger.

Chapter 5

Answers To Frequently Asked Questions

What are the CKD Complications?

Almost any part of your body can be affected by chronic kidney disease. A few of the possible complications are:

- Retention of fluid that might result in high blood pressure, pulmonary edema (build-up of fluid in the lungs) or swelling in your legs and arms.
- Anemia
- Hyperkalemia, which is an abrupt increase in the concentration of potassium in your blood. This could be detrimental to the functioning of your heart and is potentially fatal.
- Reduction in libido decreased fertility or erectile dysfunction.
- Cardiovascular disease, which affects the heart and blood vessels.
- Increased susceptibility to infections due to a reduction in immunity.
- Reduction in bone strength and higher susceptibility to the bone.
- End-stage kidney disease, which is permanent damage in the kidneys that requires renal transplant or dialysis to survive.
- Central Nervous System damage, which could impair concentration and result in seizures or personality changes.
- Pregnancy complications, which might result in risks for the growing fetus and mother.
- Pericarditis, which is an inflammation of the pericardium – the sac-like membrane that encloses the heart.

What are the Stages of CKD?

Alteration in the glomerular filtration rate (GFR) could be an indicator of the progression of kidney disease. The UK and many other countries use this method to determine the stage of kidney disease.

Stage 1: Normal GFR. Although there has been a detection of kidney disease.

Stage 2: GFR is less than 90 milliliters, and there is a detection of evidence of kidney disease

Stage 3: GFR is less than 60 milliliters, irrespective of the detection of evidence of kidney disease.

Stage 4: GFR is less than 30 milliliters, irrespective of the detection of evidence of kidney disease.

Stage 5: GFR is less than 15 milliliters. The kidney has failed. For most patients with chronic kidney disease, there is hardly a progression of kidney disease further than stage two.

Note that early diagnosis of kidney disease is important to ensure the early treatment to prevent irreversible damage. Diabetic patients should get a yearly test to detect micro albuminuria (the presence of minute quantities of protein in the urine). This test helps in the early detection of diabetic nephropathy, which is early kidney damage that is caused by diabetes.

How to Prevent CKD?

To lessen your risk of developing kidney disease:

Follow the instructions on the over-the-counter medications: When using over-the-counter pain-relieving medicines, read the instructions as contained on the label and package. Consuming too many pain relievers should be avoided since it can lead to kidney damage. Consult with your physician to find out if the drugs are suitable and safe for you.

Maintain a healthy weight: If you are currently keeping a healthy weight, try to maintain it by engaging in physical activity a greater number of days in a week. If, however, you need to reduce weight, consult your physician for the appropriate steps to take in order to reduce your weight. Normally, this calls for increasing daily physical activity and slowing down on your calorie intake.

Don't smoke: Smoking cigarettes can damage your kidney and cause your already damaged kidney to deteriorate. If you happen to be a smoker, consult with your physician about what you need to do to give up smoking. Remember that support groups, counseling, and medication can assist you to quit smoking.

Manage your medical conditions with your doctor's help: In case you have some diseases or prone to the risk of kidney disease, be close to your doctor who will help you control them. Find out from your physician the test and symptoms to watch out for to reveal the extent of your kidney damage.

How to Treat CKD?

In the meantime, there is no cure for prolonged kidney disease. But some therapies can help in controlling the signs and symptoms, slow down the disease progression, and lessen the danger of complications. Patients with prolonged kidney disease normally need to take larger doses of medications.

Chapter 6

Best Advice To Avoid Dialysis

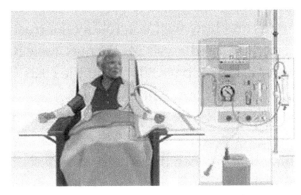

A hemodialysis treatment lasts different amounts of time because it depends on various aspects. A few examples with things that could affect the time is how well your kidneys are working, the waste and amount of it you have in your body, how big you are or the type of artificial kidney that is being used on you.

Usually however it lasts for a few hours it's done a few times a week. If you are using high flux dialysis it may take less time. The other form of dialysis is called peritoneal dialysis. This form of treatment will be having your blood cleaned inside your body. As such you will have a surgery to place a catheter into your abdomen to make an assess. During this type of treatment the area is slowly going to be filled with dialysate through the catheter and it's going to help you because the blood stays in arteries and the veins that line that cavity so the excess fluid and the waste will be drawn out of your blood and into the dialysate that's being filled through the catheter. There are two different forms of this dialysis. There is what is known as CAPD which is done without machines. You do this yourself 5 times a day. The bag of dialysate into the cavity through the catheter and remains inside for approximately 5 hours before it will drain back into the bag and then you throw away the bag. APD is the other form and it's performed using a machine called a cycler. Each cycle lasts about 90 minutes and what is known as exchanges will be performed at night when you are sleeping.

It is important to know their dialysis cannot cure this medical condition. It can do work that a healthy organ would, but it can't solve this disease completely. Though it can help your kidneys get better it's not a cure all. It can be discomforting when the needles are put into your fistula, but most patients don't have any issues. The treatment in itself is painless but you may feel sick to your stomach when you get a drop in blood pressure which can happen to some patients. If you have frequent treatments this will eventually go away. Though you can live on dialysis the rest of your life, unless a kidney transplant is in your future, the expectancy on dialysis depends on different things. It can depend on your other medical conditions and how well you follow the treatment plan. Some have been able to live for 2 or 3 decades on dialysis others may have 5 to 10. Dialysis can be expensive, but the federal government pays 80% of all the costs for patients. Another fact is that most people are able to live a normal life.

Now that we've discussed what dialysis is let's talk about how to avoid it. You can delay the onset of dialysis by eating right and losing any excess weight. You should also avoid smoking. This is a vital thing that you can do to help your body. Another thing to do is to control your blood pressure and diabetes. Junk food is a staple in mand diets, but you need to avoid excess salt in your diet and make sure that you are eating healthy.

Staying with health insurance so that you can get regularly checked out by your doctor and that you're talking to your health care team is important too. They will help to make sure that you're not having kidney issues or if you are having kidney issues to make sure that you are following their instructions perfectly so that you don't have to have dialysis. Regardless of how a person develops chronic kidney disease there are still actions that you can take to prolong having to use dialysis. The healthier you are the longer your kidneys will be able to function properly but because everyone's kidney condition is unique you'll still have to talk to your doctor and make sure that they can give you some helpful hints as well to avoid having to use dialysis.

Chapter 7

Recipes

Breakfast Recipes

Poached Eggs with Butter

*Servings: 2 / Total Time: 15 Minutes / Calories: 261 / Protein: 14 g / Sodium: 164 mg /
Potassium: 173 mg / Phosphorus: 226 mg*

Ingredients and Quantity

- Pepper, to taste
- Vinegar
- 4 eggs
- 1 tbsp. chopped cilantro
- 2 tbsp. unsalted butter
  - 1 tbsp. chopped parsley

Direction

1. Place a pan on low heat and melt the butter.

2. Add in the cilantro and parsley. Allow this to cook for around 1 minute, stirring constantly.

3. Set it off the heat and pour in a small bowl.

4. In a small pot, add 3 inches of water and allow this to come to a simmer. Add in a dash of vinegar.

5. Crack one of the eggs into a small bowl. With a spoon, swirl the water to create a whirlpool, and then slowly pour the water.

6. With your spoon, help the whites draw over the yolk of the egg. Repeat this for the rest of the eggs.

7. Allow them to cook for about 4 to 7 minutes, depending on how you want yolk to be.

8. Using a slotted spoon, take the eggs out and allow to drain for a minute.

9. Serve the eggs with a tbsp. of the herbed butter and a sprinkling of pepper. Enjoy!

Breakfast Tacos

Servings: 4 / Total Time: 15 Minutes / Calories: 210 / Protein: 9 g / Sodium: 364 mg / Potassium: 141 mg / Phosphorus: 120 mg

Ingredients and Quantity

- 1/4 cup tomato salsa
- 4 tortillas
- Red pepper flakes
- 1/2 tsp. ground cumin
- 4 eggs
- 1/2 tsp. minced garlic
- 1/2 chopped bell pepper
- 1/2 chopped sweet onion
  - **1 tsp. olive oil**

Direction

1. Warm the oil in a large pan over medium heat.

2. Place the garlic, bell pepper, and onion into the skillet, cooking until soft. This will take around 5 minutes.

3. Add in the red pepper flakes, cumin, and eggs.

4. Scramble the eggs along with the vegetables until they are cooked to your likeness.

5. Divide the eggs evenly between the 4 tortillas.

6. Top each with 1 tablespoon of salsa. Serve and enjoy!

Grapefruit in Broiled Honey

Servings: 2 / Total Time: 10 Minutes / Calories: 6 / Protein: 1 g / Sodium: 1 mg / Potassium: 175 mg / Phosphorus: 1 mg /

Ingredients and Quantity

- 1 grapefruit
- 2 tsp. honey
- 1/4 tsp. cinnamon

Direction

1. Preheat the broiler at 300 F (150 C).
2. Cut your grapefruit in half and cut it in the form of a semicircle
3. Drizzle the top of each grapefruit with honey and 1/8 teaspoon of cinnamon
4. Broil it for 6 minutes until it starts to brown and serve it hot. Enjoy!

Hash Brown Omelet

Servings: 2 / Total Time: 15 Minutes / Calories: 225 / Protein: 15 g / Sodium: 180 mg / Potassium: 305 mg / Phosphorus: 128 mg /

Ingredients and Quantity

- 2 tbsp. diced onion
- 1 tsp. canola oil
- 2 tbsp. shredded hash brown
- 2 tbsp. diced fresh green bell pepper
- 1 egg
- 2 tbsp. soy milk
- 2 egg whites
- 2 pieces parsley

Direction

1. Heat oil at medium heat and add the diced onion pieces and green pepper, cooking it for 2 minutes.
2. Add hash brown and cook it or heat it (if not frozen) for 5 minutes.
3. Meanwhile, beat the eggs with soy milk and add nondairy creamer.
4. Pour the eggs in a pan and cook them to prepare an omelet until it is ready and firm. Place the hash brown on the omelet in the middle and roll it on a plate.
5. Add parsley and spices. Serve and enjoy!

Omelet with Apple and Onion

Servings: 2 / Total Time: 20 Minutes / Calories: 284 / Protein: 13 g / Sodium: 165 mg / Potassium: 340 mg / Phosphorus: 23 mg /

Ingredients and Quantity

- 3 eggs
- 1 tbsp. water
- 1 tbsp. butter
- 1 apple
- 1/4 cup low fat milk
- 1/8 tbsp. black pepper
- 2 small spoons cheddar cheese
- 3/4 cup sweet onion

Direction

1. Peel the apple and slice thinly both apple and onion
2. Pre heat the oven at 400° F (that is around 200°C)
3. Prepare a small bowl and put in it both water, eggs with milk, pepper, and leave it there.
4. Melt the butter over medium heat. Add apple and onion and wait until the onion becomes translucent for about 5 - 6 minutes.
5. Spread the mix of onion and apple in the bowl and put the egg mixture over medium heat until the edges set. Then add cheddar over the top and put the skillet in the oven for about 10 minutes.
6. Divide the omelet into two parts and put it on a plate, serving it immediately. Enjoy!

Roll Up Burrito

Servings: 2 / Total Time: 20 Minutes / Calories: 366 / Protein: 18 g / Sodium: 590 mg / Potassium: 245 mg / Phosphorus: 300 mg /

Ingredients and Quantity

- 4 eggs
- 3 tbsp. green chilies
- 1/2 tsp. pepper sauce
- 1/4 tsp. ground cumin
- 2 flour tortillas in burrito size
- Nonstick cooking spray

Direction

1. Put the non-stick cooking spray in a pan and heat a medium heat.
2. Beat eggs with green chilies, cumin and hot pepper sauce.
3. Put the eggs into the pan and cook them for 2 minutes.
4. Heat tortillas in a skillet at medium heat.
5. Place half the eggs mix on each tortilla and roll up. Serve and enjoy!

Vanilla Waffles

Servings: 2 / Total Time: 15 Minutes / Calories: 367 / Protein: 8 g / Sodium: 200 mg / Potassium: 150 mg / Phosphorus: 120 mg /

Ingredients and Quantity

- 2 eggs
- 2 glasses cake flour
- 3/4 glass low fat milk
- 3/4 tsp. baking soda
- 3/4 cup sour cream
- 6 tbsp. powdered sugar
- 4 tbsp. unsalted butter
- 2 tsp. vanilla extract
- 2 tbsp. granulated sugar

Direction

1. Heat the waffle iron.

2. Put together the cake flour and baking soda.
3. Separate egg whites and yolks. Mix together egg yolks, sour cream, milk and vanilla.
4. Melt the butter and put it into the sour cream mix.
5. In another cup beat the egg whites with a hand mixer on medium speed until the peak is soft and add granulated sugar to the egg whites, still beating until stiff peaks form for 3 or 4 minutes.
6. Beat the sour cream mixture into the flour mix until they combine and then add the egg whites to smooth everything.
7. Add the batter to the waffle iron, close and cook for about 3-4 minutes.
8. Serve waffles with powder sugar on it or top it with fresh berries, jam, syrup or whipped cream. Enjoy!

Yogurt Fantasy

Servings: 2 / Total Time: 15 Minutes / Calories: 185 / Protein: 28 g / Sodium: 122 mg / Potassium: 334 mg / Phosphorus: 215 mg /

Ingredients and Quantity

- Greek yogurt
- 1 spoon vanilla whey protein powder
- 1/2 cup blueberries

Direction

1. Add protein powder to the yogurt slowly and mix after each addition. Do not mix all at once or it may be clumpy.
2. Wash the blueberries and dry them.
3. Place on top of the yogurt mixture. Serve and enjoy!

Feta and Bell Pepper Quiche

Servings: 5 / Total Time: 30 Minutes / Calories: 172 / Protein: 8 g / Sodium: 154 mg / Potassium: 122 mg / Phosphorus: 120 mg /

Ingredients and Quantity

- Pepper, to taste
- 2 tbsp. chopped basil
- 1/4 cup low sodium feta cheese

- 1/4 cup plain flour
- 4 eggs
- 1 cup unsweetened rice milk
- 1 chopped bell pepper
- 1 tsp. minced garlic
- 1 small chopped sweet onion
- 1 tsp. olive oil plus more

Direction

1. Warm your oven to 400 F. Brush a small amount of olive oil into a 9 inch pie pan.
2. Warm the oil in a skillet on medium heat.
3. Cook the onion and garlic until they become soft.
4. Add in bell pepper and cook for another 3 minutes.
5. Place the vegetables into the pie plate that has been brushed with olive oil.
6. Place the eggs, flour, and rice milk in a medium bowl and combine until smooth.
7. Add in the basil and feta, then sprinkle with pepper. Stir well to combine.
8. Pour eggs over the vegetables in the pie plate.
9. Bake until edges are golden brown and center is just set. This should take about 20 minutes.
10. This can be served cold, room temperature, or hot. Enjoy!

Pumpkin Apple Muffins

Servings: 12 / *Total Time:* 25 Minutes / *Calories:* 125 / *Protein:* 2 g / *Sodium:* 8 mg / *Potassium:* 177 mg / *Phosphorus:* 120 mg /

Ingredients and Quantity

- 1/2 cup diced cored and peeled apple
- 1 tsp. vanilla
- 1 egg
- 1/4 cup olive oil
- 1/4 cup honey
- 1 cup pumpkin puree
- 2 tsp. Phosphorus=free baking powder
- 1 cup wheat bran
- 1 cup plain flour

Direction

1. Warm the oven to 350 F. Take a cupcake tin and place a paper liner into each cup.
2. Add baking powder, wheat bran and flour into a medium bowl. Stir to mix well.
3. Add the vanilla, egg, olive oil, honey and pumpkin to a small bowl and combine.
4. Mix the pumpkin mixture into the dry ingredients.
5. Add in the apple and stir to combine.
6. Spoon batter into muffin papers. Don't overfill.
7. Bake for 20 minutes. Once over, stick a toothpick in the middle. If it comes out clean, it means they are done. Serve and enjoy!

Bread Pudding with Blueberries

Servings: 6 / Total Time: 25 Minutes / Calories: 382 / Protein: 11 g / Sodium: 378 mg / Potassium: 170 mg / Phosphorus: 120 mg /

Ingredients and Quantity

- 2 cups blueberries
- 6 cups sourdough bread cubes
- 1/2 tsp. ground cinnamon
- 2 tsp. vanilla
- 3 eggs
- 1/2 cup honey
- 3 cups unsweetened rice milk

Direction

1. Warm your oven to 350 F.
2. Add cinnamon, vanilla, eggs, honey, and rice milk to a large bowl until well-blended.
3. Add in the bread cubes. Allow the bread to soak for 30 minutes.
4. Add in the blueberries. Stir well to combine. Pour into a 13 x 9 baking dish.
5. Bake for 35 minutes. Check to see if it's done by poking it in the center with a toothpick and it comes out clean. Serve and enjoy!

Citrus Blueberry Muffins

Servings: 12 / Total Time: 25 Minutes / Calories: 252 / Protein: 4 g / Sodium: 26 mg / Potassium: 107 mg / Phosphorus: 79 mg /

Ingredients and Quantity

- 2 cups blueberries
- 2 tsp. phosphorus-free baking powder
- 1 tsp. lime zest
- 2 cups plain flour
- 1/2 cup light sour cream
- 1 tsp. lemon zest
- 1 cup unsweetened rice milk
- 2 eggs
- 1 cup sugar
- 1/2 cup melted coconut oil

Direction

1. Warm the oven for 400 F. Take a cupcake tin and place paper liners in each cup.
2. Place the sugar and coconut oil into a medium bowl. Using a hand mixer, beat until fluffy.
3. Add in sour cream, rice milk and eggs.
4. Scrape and continue to mix until well blended.
5. Add baking powder, lime zest, lemon zest, and flour to a small bowl. Stir together to combine.
6. Mix the flour mixture into the eggs until it just comes together. Add in the blueberries and stir again.
7. Spoon into prepared muffin papers. Don't overfill.
8. Place into the preheated oven and bake for 25 minutes.
9. Check to make sure a toothpick comes out clean when stuck to the muffins. Serve and enjoy!

Oatmeal Pancakes

Servings: 4 / Total Time: 10 Minutes / Calories: 195 / Protein: 6 g / Sodium: 60 mg / Potassium: 92 mg / Phosphorus: 109 mg /

Ingredients and Quantity

- 1 tbsp. unsalted butter, divided
- 1 egg
- 1/2 cup unsweetened rice milk
- Ground cinnamon, to taste
- 1/4 cup rolled oats
- 1 cup plain flour

Direction

1. Put cinnamon, oats and flour into a medium bowl and stir well to combine.
2. Add the egg and milk to the same bowl. Whisk together.
3. Add this to the flour mixture and whisk well to combine.
4. On a large skillet over medium heat, melt the butter.
5. Take .25 cup of the batter and pour it into the skillet.
6. Cook the pancake until edges are firm and there are bubbles on the surface. This should take about 3 minutes.
7. Flip the pancake and cook until golden brown on this side. This will take around 2 more minutes.
8. Continue with the rest of the batter until it is completely used. Add butter to skillet as needed.
9. Serve pancakes hot. Enjoy!

Asparagus Frittata

Servings: 2 / Total Time: 30 Minutes / Calories: 102 / Protein: 6 g / Sodium: 46 mg / Potassium: 248 mg / Phosphorus: 103 mg /

Ingredients and Quantity

- 1/4 cup chopped parsley
- 1/2 tsp. onion powder
- 4 eggs
- Pepper, to taste
- 2 tsp. EVOO, divided
- 10 medium trimmed asparagus spears

Direction

1. Start by placing your oven to 450 F. Toss the asparagus spears with a teaspoon of oil and season with a bit of pepper.
2. Lay these out on a cookie sheet and bake for 20 minutes. Stir the spears occasionally and allow them to cook until they are tender and browned.
3. Beat the eggs together with the parsley and onion powder. Add pepper to taste.
4. Slice the asparagus into 1-inch pieces and lay them in the bottom of a medium pan.
5. Drizzle in the remaining oil and shake the pan so that everything distributes.
6. Pour the egg mixture over the asparagus and cook them over medium heat.

7. Once the eggs have set up on the bottom and almost set on the top, place a plate and flip over the pan so that the frittata is on the plate, and then carefully slide the frittata back in the pan to cook on the other side.
8. Allow this to continue cooking for 30 more seconds, or until set. Serve and enjoy!

Broccoli Basil Quiche

Servings: 8 / Total Time: 60 Minutes / Calories: 160 / Protein: 6 g / Sodium: 259 mg / Potassium: 173 mg / Phosphorus: 101 mg /

Ingredients and Quantity

- Pepper, to taste
- 1 tbsp. all-purpose flour
- Minced garlic clove, to taste
- 1/2 cup crumbled feta
- 1 cup unsweetened rice milk
- 2 tbsp. chopped basil
- 3 eggs, beaten
- 2 chopped scallions
- Chopped tomato, to taste
- 2 cup finely chopped broccoli
- 1 frozen pie crust

Direction

1. Turn your oven to 425 F.
2. Lay the pie crust out into a pan and use a fork to pierce the crust in a few places so that it doesn't rise too much.
3. Allow the crust to bake for about 10 minutes.
4. Remove and lower the temperature of the oven to 325° F.
5. In a medium bowl, combine the flour, garlic, feta, rice milk, basil, eggs, scallions, tomato, and broccoli. Sprinkle in some pepper.
6. Pour the egg mixture into the pie crust. Allow this to bake for 35 to 45 minutes. When you insert a knife in the center, it should come out clean.
7. Allow the quiche to cool for 10 to 15 minutes before you serve. Enjoy!

Avocado Egg Bake

Servings: 2 / *Total Time:* 20 Minutes / *Calories:* 242 / *Protein:* 9 g / *Sodium:* 88 mg / *Potassium:* 575 mg / *Phosphorus:* 164 mg /

Ingredients and Quantity

- 1 tbsp. chopped parsley
- Pepper, to taste
- 2 eggs
- Halved avocado

Direction

1. Start by placing the oven to 425 F.
2. Carefully crack one egg in a small bowl, making sure that the yolk doesn't break.
3. Lay the avocado halves on a baking sheet with the cut side up. Pour the egg into the center of one of the avocado halves.
4. Repeat this for the other egg and other avocado half. Sprinkle with some pepper.
5. Bake for 15 minutes or until the eggs are set to your desired doneness.
6. Remove and sprinkle with the parsley before serving. Enjoy!

Lunch

Mexican Beef Flour Wrap

Servings: 2 / *Total Time:* 10 Minutes / *Calories:* 255 / *Protein:* 24 g / *Sodium:* 275 mg / *Potassium:* 445 mg / *Phosphorus:* 250 mg /

Ingredients and Quantity

- 5 oz. cooked roast beef
- 8 cucumber slices
- 2 flour tortillas, 6 inch size
- 2 tbsp. whipped cream cheese
- 2 leaves light green lettuce
- 1/4 bowl cut red onion
- 1/4 stripped cut sweet bell pepper
- 1 tsp. herb seasoning blend

Direction

1. Spread the cheese over the flour wraps. Try to use the ingredients to make two wraps.
2. Layer the tortillas with roast beef, onions, lettuce, pepper strips and cucumber.
3. Sprinkle with the herb seasoning.
4. Roll up the wraps and cut them into 4 pieces each. Serve fresh. Enjoy!

Mixed Chorizo in Egg Flour Wraps

Servings: 2 / *Total Time:* 10 Minutes / *Calories:* 223 / *Protein:* 15 g / *Sodium:* 315 mg / *Potassium:* 285 mg / *Phosphorus:* 230 mg /

Ingredients and Quantity

- 1 pack chorizo
- 1 egg
- 1 flour tortilla or 6 inch size

Direction

1. Cook the chorizo in a pan on stove, cutting the meat into small pieces.
2. Eliminate excessive water or fat and add 1 egg combining all while they are being cooked.
3. Serve everything on a flour tortilla or wrapping the tortillas. Enjoy!

Sandwich with Chicken Salad

Servings: 2 / Total Time: 10 Minutes / Calories: 345 / Protein: 22 g / Sodium: 395 mg / Potassium: 330 mg / Phosphorus: 165 mg /

Ingredients and Quantity

- 2 bowls cooked chicken
- 1/2 cup low-fat mayonnaise
- 1/2 cup green bell pepper
- 1 cup pieces pineapple
- 1/3 cup carrots
- 4 slices flatbread
- 1/2 tsp. black pepper

Direction

1. Prepare aside the diced chicken and drain pineapple, adding green bell pepper, black pepper and carrots.
2. Combine all in a bowl and refrigerate until chilled.
3. Later on, serve the chicken salad on the flatbread. Enjoy!

Spice Bread with Tuna Salad

Servings: 2 / Total Time: 10 Minutes / Calories: 290 / Protein: 25 g / Sodium: 475 mg / Potassium: 320 mg / Phosphorus: 175 mg /

Ingredients and Quantity

- 1 tbsp. onion
- 1 piece celery
- 1 fresh tomato
- Some lettuce leaves
- 1 tbsp. low calories mayonnaise

- 1 medium bagel or spiced bread
- 1/2 pack low sodium water-packed canned tuna

Direction

1. Chop onion, tomato and celery.
2. Open tuna and cut into small pieces.
3. Put everything in the bagel on the lettuce leaves, adding some mayonnaise and then close the bread. Serve and enjoy!

Tiny Rice Pies

Servings: 2 / Total Time: 10 Minutes / Calories: 175 / Protein: 5 g / Sodium: 214 mg / Potassium: 140 mg / Phosphorus: 89 mg /

Ingredients and Quantity

- 2 tbsp. vegetable oil
- 1 tsp. mustard seeds
- 1/2 cup semolina
- 2 green finely cut chilies
- 1/8 tsp. salt
- 1/4 cup yogurt
- 1/4 glass water
- 1/4 grated corn
- 1/4 Indian cheese
- Some bits finely cut cilantro
- 1 tbsp. clarified butter

Direction

1. Heat the oil and the seeds in a pan and add semolina, chilies and a bit of salt.
2. Cook it until the semolina becomes a bit brown. Let it cool down. Put together yogurt with some water and mix it until it is smooth, then add corn, Indian cheese, cilantro, yogurt and add everything to semolina, leaving it aside for 10-15 minutes.
3. Put the clarified butter in a pan, steaming then the semolina mix for 10 minutes.
4. Put some cilantro on the semolina circles and serve them still a bit warm. Enjoy!

Toast Topped with Creamy Eggs

Servings: 2 / Total Time: 15 Minutes / Calories: 430 / Protein: 15 g / Sodium: 400 mg / Potassium: 250 mg / Phosphorus: 210 mg /

Ingredients and Quantity

- 4 slices white bread
- 6 eggs
- 4 oz. cream cheese
- 3 tbsp. unsalted butter
- 1/3 cup flour
- 1 1/2 cups unsweetened, plain almond milk
- 1/2 tbsp. yellow mustard
- 1/8 tsp. pepper

Direction

1. Hard boil the eggs for 12 minutes. Remove them from heat, drain and cover with cool water.
2. Peel and chop boiled eggs. Put together the butter and flour in a sauce pan at medium low heat.
3. Mix constantly until well combined.
4. Add almond milk, cream cheese, mustard and pepper to butter and flour mixture. Let it thicken and add the eggs to the sauce, keeping at a warm heat.
5. Toast the bread and put the egg mixture over the toast before serving. Enjoy!

Fresh Cucumber Soup

Servings: 2 / Total Time: 2 Hours 5 Minutes / Calories: 78 / Protein: 2 g / Sodium: 127 mg / Potassium: 257 mg / Phosphorus: 65 mg /

Ingredients and Quantity

- 2 cucumbers
- 1/3 cup white onion
- 1 green onion
- 1/4 cup fresh mint
- 2 tbsp. fresh lemon juice
- 2 tbsp. fresh dill
- 2/3 cup water

- 1/3 cup sour cream
- 1/2 cup half and half cream
- 1/2 tsp. pepper
- 1/4 tsp. salt

Direction

1. Remove both peel and seeds from cucumbers.
2. Cut mint and the onions. Cut up dill.
3. Put all ingredients in a mixer and whisk until smooth.
4. Cover and place in the refrigerator for at least 2 hour.
5. Use fresh dill sprigs to garnish the soup. Serve and enjoy!

Berry Salad with Italian Ricotta Cheese

Servings: 2 / Total Time: 5 Minutes / Calories: 140 / Protein: 15 g / Sodium: 380 mg / Potassium: 350 mg / Phosphorus: 180 mg /

Ingredients and Quantity

- 1 cup fresh blackberries
- 1 cup fresh blueberries
- 2 cups fresh strawberries
- 1/3 cup lemon juice
- 2 cups fresh Italian ricotta cheese
- 1/8 tsp. cinnamon

Direction

1. Wash well both blackberries and blueberries and strawberries. Slice them and put them all together.
2. Add some lemon juice from the cup.
3. Put the ricotta cheese on a round plate or a bowl and then cover it with berries.
4. Spread the cinnamon on it. Serve and enjoy!

Celery Tuna Salad

Servings: 2 / Total Time: 5 Minutes / Calories: 20 / Protein: 15 g / Sodium: 185 mg / Potassium: 318 mg / Phosphorus: 183 mg /

Ingredients and Quantity

- 1 piece celery
- 15 oz. packed and unsalted tuna
- 1/2 apple
- 1/2 small onion
- 2 tbsp. mayonnaise
- A bit of black pepper
- Pinch salt

Direction

1. Prepare the tuna and cut the apple, celery and onion.
2. Mix all together, adding mayonnaise, black pepper and if you wish, some salt.
3. Serve on lettuce and with unsalted crackers. Enjoy!

Meat Casserole

*Servings: 2 / **Total Time:** 60 Minutes / **Calories:** 222 / **Protein:** 10 g / **Sodium:** 355 mg / **Potassium:** 200 mg / **Phosphorus:** 156 mg /*

Ingredients and Quantity

- 10 oz. reduced-fat pork sausage
- 8 oz. cream cheese
- 1 glass low-fat milk
- 4 slices white bread
- 5 eggs
- 1/2 tsp. dry mustard
- 1/2 dry onion flakes

Direction

1. Preheat oven at 325°F (160°C).
2. Cut the sausage and cook in a cooking dish. Set aside and mix all other ingredients.
3. Add cooked sausage to mixture and place bread pieces in a square casserole, pour sausage mix over the bread and cook for 50 minutes.
4. Cut into 10 portions and serve. Enjoy!

Ground Beef in a Cup

Servings: 2 / *Total Time:* 10 Minutes / *Calories:* 250 / *Protein:* 25 g / *Sodium:* 160 mg / *Potassium:* 395 mg / *Phosphorus:* 245 mg /

Ingredients and Quantity

- 1/4 pound ground beef
- 2 tbsp. low fat milk
- 2 tsp. ketchup
- 2 tbsp. quick-cooked oats
- 1 tsp. onion powder

Direction

1. Spray a large cup with non-stick cooking spray.
2. In another cup put together the milk (or its substitute), ketchup, onion, oats.
3. Crumble meat over the mixture and mix everything, pressing the ground beef.
4. Cover and put it in the microwave for 3 minutes (high) and serve it very warm. Enjoy!

Dinner

Salad with Strawberries and Goat Cheese

Servings: 2 / Total Time: 15 Minutes / Calories: 300 / Protein: 13 g / Sodium: 285 mg / Potassium: 400 mg / Phosphorus: 193 mg /

Ingredients and Quantity

- Baby lettuce, to taste
- 1 pint strawberries
- Balsamic vinegar
- Extra virgin olive oil
- 1/4 tsp. black pepper
- 8 oz. soft goat cheese

Direction

1. Prepare the lettuce by washing and drying it, then cut the strawberries.
2. Cut the soft goat cheese into 8 pieces.
3. Put together the balsamic vinegar and the extra virgin olive oil in a large cup with a whisk.
4. Mix the strawberries pressing them and putting them in a bowl, add the dressing and mix, then divide the lettuce into four dishes and cut the other strawberries, arranging them on the salad.
5. Put cheese slices on top and add pepper. Serve and enjoy!

Salmon with Spicy Honey

Servings: 2 / Total Time: 15 Minutes / Calories: 320 / Protein: 23 g / Sodium: 65 mg / Potassium: 450 mg / Phosphorus: 250 mg /

Ingredients and Quantity

- 16 oz. salmon fillet

- 3 tbsp. honey
- 3/4 tsp. lemon peel
- 3 bowls arugula salad
- 1/2 tsp. black pepper
- 1/2 tsp. garlic powder
- 2 tsp. olive oil
- 1 tsp. hot water

Direction

1. Prepare a small bowl with some hot water and put in honey, grated lemon peel, ground pepper, and garlic powder.
2. Spread the mixture over salmon fillets.
3. Warm some olive oil at a medium heat and add spiced salmon fillet and cook for 4 minutes.
4. Turn the fillets on one side then on the other side.
5. Continue to cook for other 4 minutes at a reduced heat and try to check when the salmon fillets flake easily.
6. Put some arugula on each plate and add the salmon fillets on top, adding some aromatic herbs or some dill. Serve and enjoy!

Stuffed Peppers

Servings: 2 / *Total Time:* 1 Hour 15 Minutes / *Calories:* 260 / *Protein:* 20 g / *Sodium:* 210 mg / *Potassium:* 550 mg / *Phosphorus:* **208 mg** /

Ingredients and Quantity

- 4 bell peppers
- 1 tbsp. dried parsley
- 2 cups cooked white rice
- 2 tsp. garlic powder
- 1 tsp. black pepper
- 3/4 pound ground beef
- 1/2 bowl chopped onion
- 3 oz. unsalted tomato sauce

Direction

1. Remove the seeds from black peppers
2. Preheat the oven at 375°F (or 200°C)

3. Roast the beef and add onion, rice, parsley, black pepper, garlic powder and tomato sauce to the beef.
4. Boil slowly for 10 minutes.
5. Feel the bell peppers with mixture and bake in the oven for one hour. Serve and enjoy!

Turkey Sausages

Servings: 2 / Total Time: 10 Minutes / Calories: 55 / Protein: 7 g / Sodium: 70 mg / Potassium: 105 mg / Phosphorus: 75 mg /

Ingredients and Quantity

- 1/4 tsp. salt
- 1/8 tsp. garlic powder
- 1/8 tsp. onion powder
- 1 tsp. fennel seed
- 1 pound 7% fat ground turkey

Direction

1. Press the fennel seed and in a small cup put together turkey with fennel seed, garlic and onion powder and salt.
2. Cover the bowl and refrigerate overnight.
3. Prepare the turkey with seasoning into different portions with a circle form and press them into patties ready to be cooked.
4. Cook at a medium heat until browned.
5. Cook it for 1 to 2 minutes per side and serve them hot. Enjoy!

Zucchini and Carrots Rosemary Chicken

Servings: 2 / Total Time: 10 Minutes / Calories: 215 / Protein: 28 g / Sodium: 105 mg / Potassium: 580 mg / Phosphorus: 250 mg /

Ingredients and Quantity

- 2 zucchini
- 1 carrot
- 1 tsp. dried rosemary
- 4 chicken breasts
- 1/2 bell pepper

- 1/2 red onion
- 8 garlic cloves
- Olive oil
- 1/4 tbsp. ground pepper

Direction

1. Prepare the oven and preheat it at 375 °F (or 200°C).
2. Slice both zucchini and carrots and add bell pepper, onion, garlic and put everything adding oil in a 13" x 9" pan.
3. Spread the pepper over everything and roast for about 10 minutes.
4. Meanwhile, lift up the chicken skin and spread black pepper and rosemary on the flesh.
5. Remove the vegetable pan from the oven and add the chicken, returning the pan to the oven for about 30 more minutes. Serve and enjoy!

Ground Beef Soup

Servings: 2 / Total Time: 1 Hour 15 Minutes / Calories: 220 / Protein: 20 g / Sodium: 170 mg / Potassium: 445 mg / Phosphorus: 210 mg /

Ingredients and Quantity

- 1 pound lean ground beef, cut into small balls
- 1/2 glass onion
- 1 small spoon seasoning and browning sauce
- 2 small spoons lemon pepper seasoning blend
- Some low sodium beef consommé
- 2 glasses water
- 1/2 dish white rice
- 1/2 pack frozen mixed vegetables (corn, carrots, peas, beans and green beans)
- 1/2 tsp. sour cream

Direction

1. Brown ground beef with cut onion in a pan and eliminate fat. Add seasoning sauce, water, consommé, rice and vegetables.
2. On high heat, boil the ingredients and after lowering the heat, cook for 30 minutes.
3. Put the meatballs in the consommé and cook at a low heat still for half an hour until ready to serve. Enjoy!

Ground Turkey Burger

Servings: 2 / Total Time: 15 Minutes / Calories: 28 / Protein: 24 g / Sodium: 285 mg / Potassium: 510 mg / Phosphorus: 235 mg /

Ingredients and Quantity

- 1 pound ground lean turkey
- 6 hamburger buns
- 1/2 dish red onion
- 1/2 dish green bell pepper
- 1/2 spoon chicken grilled blend seasoning
- 2 tsp. brown sugar
- 1 tbsp. Worcestershire sauce
- 1 cup low sodium tomato sauce

Direction

1. Cook the turkey at medium heat.
2. Cut little pieces of onion and green bell pepper.
3. Mix the sauce, the grilled blend seasoning and tomato sauce.
4. Add seasoning to the turkey mixture and cook for 10 minutes.
5. Prepare 5 portions and put in burger buns. Serve and enjoy!

One Portion Frittatas

Servings: 2 / Total Time: 45 Minutes / Calories: 110 / Protein: 8 g / Sodium: 115 mg / Potassium: 160 mg / Phosphorus: 130 mg /

Ingredients and Quantity

- 4 eggs
- 2 tsp. red bell pepper
- 2 tbsp. green bell pepper
- 2 tbsp. onion
- 2 oz. cooked lean ham
- 1 tbsp. low fat milk
- 1 pound frozen hash brown potatoes
- 1/2 bowl low fat cheddar cheese
- Black pepper

Direction

1. Put the potatoes in water in a bowl for 4 hours. Eliminate excessive water.
2. Pre heat oven at 375°F (or 200°C).
3. Coat 8 muffin tins holes with cooking spray. Put hash brown potatoes in the tins and press them in the bottom then spray also the potatoes with cooking spray.
4. Cook for 12-15 minutes at 350°F (175° C).
5. Cut the ham, pepper and onion finely and beat both milk and eggs together in a bowl.
6. Season with pepper and add ham, pepper, onion and cheese to the mixture. Enjoy!
7. Put the hash brown potatoes in the muffin holes pressing them and out ¼ bowl egg mixture in the center of each muffin hole. Put again the pan in the oven and let the potatoes become crispy in about 15 to 20 minutes.
8. Once ready, let the muffins sit on a dish for 5 minutes before serving. Enjoy!

Pan Fried Beef and Broccoli

Servings: 2 / Total Time: 25 Minutes / Calories: 370 / Protein: 18 g / Sodium: 350 mg / Potassium: 550 mg / Phosphorus: 250 mg /

Ingredients and Quantity

- 2 garlic small slices
- 1 tomato
- 8 oz. uncooked lean sirloin beef
- 12 oz. frozen broccoli stir fry vegetable blend
- 2 little spoons peanut oil
- 1/4 cup low sodium chicken consommé
- 1 tsp. cornstarch
- 2 tsp. low sodium soy sauce
- 2 bowls cooked rice

Direction

1. Cut the garlic cloves and tomato.
2. Cut the beef into strips and place the broccoli in the microwave for 3-4 minutes.
3. In a wok pan heat oil and the garlic to make them fragrant. Add vegetable blend cooking it for about 4 minutes or more and remove from pan.
4. Add the beef in the same pot and cook it for around 7-8 minutes, then prepare the sauce putting together the consommé, the soy sauce and cornstarch.
5. Add vegetables, sauce, tomato and heat them with the beef until the sauce is ready.

6. Serve the dish with brown rice. Enjoy!

Pork Chops and Apples

Servings: 2 / Total Time: 45 Minutes / Calories: 490 / Protein: 25 g / Sodium: 365 mg / Potassium: 405 mg / Phosphorus: 220 mg /

Ingredients and Quantity

- 2 tbsp. unsalted margarine
- 6 oz. low sodium stuffing mix for chicken
- 20 oz. apple pie filling
- 6 boneless pork loin chops
- Olive oil

Direction

1. Put a baking pan in the oven at 350°F (or 200°C) and grease it with olive oil.
2. Put together the stuffing and mix it in water and margarine. Spread the apple pie pieces on the bottom of the pan and place pork chops on it.
3. Put the stuffing on top of pork chops.
4. Cover with parchment paper and bake for 30 minutes.
5. Remove the paper and still leave it in the oven for 10 minutes. Serve and enjoy!

Rigatoni Spring Pasta

Servings: 2 / Total Time: 20 Minutes / Calories: 253 / Protein: 10 g / Sodium: 115 mg / Potassium: 250 mg / Phosphorus: 153 mg /

Ingredients and Quantity

- 12 oz. rigatoni pasta (you can also use fusilli or farfalle pasta)
- 12 oz. vegetables (carrots, broccoli and zucchini or any other fresh vegetable)
- 2 portions half and half creamer
- Grated parmesan cheese

Direction

1. Boil the water and when the water starts producing bubbles, put the pasta in it. For Rigatoni it will take around 11 minutes to cook. In the meantime put the cut and diced

vegetables into a pan with some olive oil in it. Mix the vegetables until they are soft and ready, adding the two small portions of half and half creamer.

2. When the pasta boils, drain it in a strainer and put it in the pan where you have prepared the vegetables.

3. Mix everything together and put the pasta on a dish, adding some parmesan cheese on top. (If you prefer you can add the parmesan cheese when you are mixing the ingredients in the pan at a medium heat).

4. Then serve hot. Enjoy!

Desserts

Pudding Glass with Banana and Whipped Cream

Servings: 2 / Total Time: 2 Hours 10 Minutes / Calories: 255 / Protein: 3 g / Sodium: 275 mg / Potassium: 50 mg / Phosphorus: 40 mg /

Ingredients and Quantity

- 2 portions banana cream pudding mix
- 2 1/2 cups rice milk
- 8 oz. dairy whipped cream
- 12 oz. vanilla wafers

Direction

1. Put vanilla wafers in a pan and in another bowl mix together banana cream pudding and rice milk.
2. Boil the ingredients blending them slowly.
3. Pour the mixture over the wafers and make 2 or 3 layers.
4. Put the pan in the fridge for one hour and afterward spread the whipped topping over the dessert.
5. Put it back in the fridge for 2 hours and serve it cool in transparent glasses. Serve and enjoy!

Chocolate Beet Cake

Servings: 12 / Total Time: 60 Minutes / Calories: 270 / Protein: 6 g / Sodium: 109 mg / Potassium: 299 mg / Phosphorus: 111 mg /

Ingredients and Quantity

- 3 cups grated beets
- 1/4 cup canola oil
- 4 eggs

- 4 oz. unsweetened chocolate
- 2 tsp. Phosphorus-free baking powder
- 2 cups all-purpose flour
- 1 cup sugar

Direction

1. Set your oven to 325 F. Grease two 8 inch cake pans.
2. Mix the baking powder, flour and sugar together. Set aside.
3. Chop up the chocolate as finely as you can and melt using a double boiler. A microwave can also be used but don't let it burn.
4. Allow it to cool and then mix in the oil and eggs.
5. Mix all of the wet ingredients into the flour mixture and combine everything together until well mixed.
6. Fold the beets in and pour the batter in the cake pans.
7. Let them bake for 40 to 50 minutes. To know it's done, the toothpick should come out clean when inserted to the cake.
8. Remove from the oven and allow them to cool.
9. Once cool, invert over a plate to remove.
10. This is great when served with whipped cream and fresh berries. Enjoy!

Strawberry Pie

Servings: 8 / Total Time: 3 Hours 25 Minutes / Calories: 265 / Protein: 3 g / Sodium: 143 mg / Potassium: 183 mg / Phosphorus: 44 mg /

Ingredients and Quantity

For the Crust:

- 1 1/2 cups Graham cracker crumbs
- 5 tbsp. unsalted butter, at room temperature
- 2 tbsp. sugar

For the Pie:

- 1 1/2 tsp. gelatin powder
- 3 tbsp. cornstarch
- 3/4 cup sugar
- 5 cups sliced strawberries, divided
- 1 cup water

Direction

1. For the crust: heat your oven to 375 F. Grease a pie pan.
2. Combine the butter, crumbs and sugar together and then press them into your pie pan.
3. Bake the crust for 10 to 15 minutes, until lightly browned.
4. Take out of the oven and let it cool completely.
5. For the pie: crush up a cup of strawberries.
6. Using a small pot, combine the sugar, water, gelatin, and cornstarch.
7. Bring the mixture in the pot up to a boil, lower the heat, and simmer until it has thickened.
8. Add in the crushed strawberries in the pot and let it simmer for another 5 minutes until the sauce has thickened up again.
9. Set it off the heat and pour into a bowl.
10. Cool until it comes to room temperature.
11. Toss the remaining berries with the sauce so that it is well distributed and pour into the pie crust and spread it out into an even layer.
12. Refrigerate the pie until cold. This will take about 3 hours. Serve and enjoy!

Grape Skillet Galette

Servings: 6 / Total Time: 2 Hours 50 Minutes / Calories: 172 / Protein: 2 g / Sodium: 65 mg / Potassium: 69 mg / Phosphorus: 21 mg /

Ingredients and Quantity

For the Crust:

- 1/2 cup unsweetened rice milk
- 4 tbsp. cold butter
- 1 tbsp. sugar
- 1 cup all-purpose flour

For the Galette:

- 1 tbsp. cornstarch
- 1/3 cup sugar
- 1 egg white
- 2 cups halved seedless grapes

Direction

1. For the crust: add the sugar and the flour to a food processor and mix for a few seconds.
2. Place in the butter and pulse until it looks like a coarse meal.

3. Add in the rice milk and combine until the dough forms.
4. Place the dough on a clean surface and shape into a disc.
5. Wrap it with a plastic wrap and place it in the fridge for 2 hours.
6. For the galette: set your oven to 425 F.
7. Mix the cornstarch and sugar and toss the grapes in.
8. Unwrap the dough and roll out on a floured surface.
9. Press it into a 14-inch circle and place in a cast iron skillet.
10. Add the grape filling in the center and spread out to fill, leaving a 2-inch crust. Fold the edge over.
11. Brush the crust with egg white and cook for 20 to 25 minutes. The crust should be golden.
12. Allow to rest for 20 minutes before you serve. Enjoy!

Pumpkin Cheesecake

Servings: 2 / Total Time: 70 Minutes / Calories: 364 / Protein: 5 g / Sodium: 245 mg / Potassium: 125 mg / Phosphorus: 65 mg /

Ingredients and Quantity

- 1 egg white
- 1 wafer crumb, 9 inch pie crust
- 1/2 small bowl of granular sugar
- 1 tsp. vanilla extract
- 1 tsp. pumpkin pie flavoring
- 1/2 bowl pumpkin cream
- 1/2 small bowl liquid egg substitute
- 8 tbsp. frozen topping, for desserts
- 16 oz. cream cheese

Direction

1. Brush pie crust with egg white and cook for 5 minutes in a preheated oven from 375°F from 375°F now down to 350°F.
2. In a large cup put together sugar, vanilla and cream cheese, beating with a mixer until smooth.
3. Beat the egg substitute and add pumpkin cream with pie flavoring: blend everything until softened.
4. Put the pumpkin mixture in a pie shell and bake for 50 minutes to set the center.
5. Then let the pie cool down and then put it in the fridge. When you wish to, serve it in 8 slices putting some topping on it. Serve and enjoy!

Small Chocolate Cakes

Servings: 2 / Total Time: 10 Minutes / Calories: 95 / Protein: 1 g / Sodium: 162 mg / Potassium: 15 mg / Phosphorus: 80 mg /

Ingredients and Quantity

- 1 box angel food cake mix
- 1 box lemon cake mix
- Water
- Nonstick cooking spray or batter
- Dark chocolate small squared chops and chocolate powder

Direction

1. Use a transparent kitchen cooking bag and put inside both lemon cake mix, angel food mix and chocolate chops.
2. Mix everything together and add water to prepare a small cupcake.
3. Put the mix in a mold to prepare a cupcake containing the ingredients and put in microwave for one-minute high temperature.
4. Slip the cupcake out of the mold and put it on a dish, let it cool and put some more chocolate crumbs on it. Serve and enjoy!

Strawberry Whipped Cream Cake

Servings: 2 / Total Time: 30 Minutes / Calories: 355 / Protein: 4 g / Sodium: 275 mg / Potassium: 145 mg / Phosphorus: 145 mg /

Ingredients and Quantity

- 1 pint whipping cream
- 2 tbsp. gelatin
- 1/2 glass cold water
- 1 glass boiling water
- 3 tbsp. lemon juice
- 1 orange glass juice
- 1 orange glass juice
- 1 tsp. sugar
- 3/4 cup sliced strawberries
- 1 large angel food cake or light sponge cake

Direction

1. Put the gelatin in cold water then add hot water and blend. Add orange and lemon juice, also add some sugar and go on blending.
2. Refrigerate and leave it there until you see it is starting to gel.
3. Whip half portion of cream and add it to the mixture along with strawberries, put wax paper in the bowl and cut the cake in small pieces.
4. In between the pieces, add the whipped cream and put everything in the fridge for one night.
5. When you take out the cake, add some whipped cream on top and decorate with some more fruit. Serve and enjoy!

Sweet Cracker Pie Crust

Servings: 2 / Total Time: 15 Minutes / Calories: 205 / Protein: 2 g / Sodium: 208 mg / Potassium: 67 mg / Phosphorus: 22 mg /

Ingredients and Quantity

- 1 bowl gelatin cracker crumbs
- 1/4 small cup sugar
- Unsalted butter

Direction

1. Mix sweet cracker crumbs, butter and sugar.
2. Put in the over preheat at 375°F.
3. Bake for 7 minutes putting it in a greased pie.
4. Let the pie cool before adding any kind of filling. Serve and enjoy!

Apple Oatmeal Crunchy

Servings: 2 / Total Time: 40 Minutes / Calories: 295 / Protein: 3 g / Sodium: 95 mg / Potassium: 190 mg / Phosphorus: 73 mg /

Ingredients and Quantity

- 5 green apples
- 1 bowl oatmeal
- A small cup brown sugar

- 1/2 cup flour
- 1 tsp. cinnamon
- 1/2 bowl butter

Direction

1. Prepare apples by cutting them in tiny slices and preheat the oven at 350°F.
2. In a cup mix oatmeal, flour, cinnamon and brown sugar.
3. Put butter in the batter and place sliced apple in a baking pan (9" x 13").
4. Spread oatmeal mix over the apples and bake for 35 minutes. Serve and enjoy!

Berry Ice Cream

Servings: 2 / Total Time: 65 Minutes / Calories: 175 / Protein: 3 g / Sodium: 95 mg / Potassium: 80 mg / Phosphorus: 40 mg /

Ingredients and Quantity

- 6 ice cream cones
- 1 cup whipped topping
- 1 cup fresh blueberries
- 4 oz. cream cheese
- 1/4 cup blueberry jam

Direction

1. Put the cream cheese in a large cup and beat it with a mixer until it is fluffy.
2. Mix with fruit and jam and whipped topping.
3. Put the mixture on the small ice cream cones and refrigerate them in the freezer for 1 hour or more until they are ready to serve. Enjoy!

Conclusion

Who says that making healthy and delicious meals for those who have kidney disease means serving only bland and same old dishes?

The information contained in this book lets you be creative with your dishes without sacrificing your health. The recipes found here are almost with no salt added, just pure flavor that come from all-natural ingredients. Should there be some not-so suitable food for people with kidney disease, it is advised that you take them in small amounts and not very often.

I hope this book was able to help you find easy-to-follow, delicious, and nutritious recipes that you can try at home and serve for your loved one or s friend with kidney disease. These recipes use mostly whole, organic, and fresh ingredients that are naturally flavorful, and nutrient-packed.

CPSIA information can be obtained
at www.ICGtesting.com
Printed in the USA
BVHW050208310321
603712BV00008B/945